NURSE STAFFING AND PATIENT CLASSIFICATION

Strategies for Success

Elizabeth Nancy Lewis, R.N., B.S., M.S., Ph.D.
Doctors Hospital of Pinole
Pinole, California

Patricia Vince Carini, R.N., B.S.N., M.P.A.
Doctors Hospital of Pinole
Pinole, California

AN ASPEN PUBLICATION®
Aspen Systems Corporation
Rockville, Maryland
Royal Tunbridge Wells
1984

Library of Congress Cataloging in Publication Data

Lewis, Elizabeth Nancy.
Nurse staffing and patient classification.

Includes index and bibliographies.
1. Nurses—Employment. 2. Hospital patients—Classification.
3. Hospitals—Staff. I. Carini, Patricia Vince. II. Title.
[DNLM: 1. Nursing staff, Hospital—Organization and administration. 2. Patients—Classification—Nursing texts.
3. Patient care planning—Organization—Nursing texts.
WY 105 L673n]
RT86.7.L48 1984 362.1'73'068 83-17246
ISBN: 0-89443-943-X

Publisher: John Marozsan
Editorial Director: Darlene Como
Executive Managing Editor: Margot Raphael
Editorial Services: Martha Sasser
Printing and Manufacturing: Debbie Collins

Library of Congress Catalog Card Number: 83-17246
ISBN: 0-89443-943-X

Printed in the United States of America

1 2 3 4 5

For Baron Richard, Bentley Sue, and Samantha Von Less, who accepted the remodeling of the castle for this book;
For Everett Anderson, who encouraged a young author long ago;
For my colleagues who have been an inspiration in making the concepts in this book reality;
For my mother, Elsie Hegman, who keeps believing in me; and
In memory of my father, Clyde Hegman, who shared my visions of success.

Elizabeth Nancy Lewis

For my husband, Mike, whose patience and understanding enhanced this endeavor;
For my parents, Bill and Mary, whose interest and enthusiasm always made this adventure worthwhile; and
For my brother, Bill, and his family, Ginger and Christopher, for their subtle contributions and comic relief during the preparation of this manuscript.

Patricia Vince Carini

Table of Contents

Preface

Nurse staffing and patient classification systems are as numerous and complex as the individuals who use them. But they can be analyzed and simplified. If those who develop a staffing system based on patient classifications have a general understanding of the basic principles of nurse staffing, of the characteristics of patient classification systems, and of the most critical factor in the nursing department—the staff nurse and the supervisor nurse—a staffing system based on patient classifications need not be a complicated maze of paper work and figures.

Our attempts to develop a workable staffing system involved a trial-and-error process, an important part of the ultimate success of our system. By talking to others in nursing management who had used systems that had either failed or were poor substitutes for a previous method, we learned that our trials and errors were not unique. Other nursing administrators and nursing management staffs were also attempting to reinvent the wheel. We also learned that each hospital is indeed unique in significant ways: the service provided, census maintained, operating budgets allotted for staffing the varieties of patients and diagnoses, the mix of professional personnel available, and the equally numerous approaches to the delivery of care. To make this book useful we had to show how our nurse staffing system based on patient classifications can be adapted to a variety of settings.

The hospital for which we developed our system, and where we are employed, is a 137-bed acute-care facility in the San Francisco Bay area. As we developed our staffing system and it began to work, other facilities became interested in using some of our principles to enhance their own system. At a number of lengthy meetings, the topic of staffing systems based on patient acuity was discussed repeatedly, often with seemingly little accomplished. Nursing administrators commented on other obstacles, such as "But our hospital is different. Your facility has mostly licensed personnel—RNs and LVNs—while I have many nursing assistants." Another nursing administrator stated, "But you're doing total care. I cannot go to total care now, even if I wanted to. With the variety of levels of personnel on my staff, I have to do team care." Still another nursing leader added,

"But we have different services than you . . . and my outpatient surgery unit is counted in my med-surg nursing hours . . . and then there's my burn unit. . . ."

The more we heard others explain why it wouldn't work, the more we believed that if our system worked for us, it could work for nursing departments in other hospitals. This book does not describe the only system that works or necessarily the best system for other facilities. Rather, the purpose of this book is to present a staffing system that, if properly implemented, can work with accepted methods of nursing care delivery. Under the delivery systems of primary care, total care, team care, and functional care, realistic nursing goal hours can be met.

We describe how our system works for us and how it functions effectively to meet a number of our facility's goals. While we do not suggest that our system is definitive, we hope to share some viable alternatives to nurse staffing systems using patient classification from which other nursing administrations may draw.

The success of any new system is greatly contingent on how the system is introduced and how change is accepted by those affected by it. Thus we have detailed the change process, particularly as it relates to the profession of nursing. People often feel threatened by change; we have tried to emphasize the importance of involving individuals and groups in the change process rather than "forcing" it on them.

Other issues deal with accountability, autonomy, and decentralization in a nursing department. These issues are crucial for developing an effective staffing system; they set the stage for planning, developing, implementing, and evaluating a staffing system.

Another purpose of this book is to stimulate some positive change toward the traditional roles of the nurse, the physician, and the hospital management team. The nursing profession is experiencing greater and more dramatic changes than during any other time. If, as nursing administrators, we are to establish our credibility and develop autonomy, we must willingly assume responsibility and accountability for the management of nursing services. We must speak out loudly enough to be heard by those individuals who for years have relied on our input and have the greatest impact on the outcome of our services and our successes, that is, physicians, hospital administrators, and hospital financial controllers. We must influence these powerful groups of individuals who have often dictated our direction and mandated our management design. As nursing administrators we must learn to take risks in order to achieve a level of autonomy.

In Chapter 6 we discuss the changing roles of, and relationships between, nursing administration, medical staff, and hospital administration. We hope that this discussion will encourage the reader to consider the role of the nurse and the profession for the 1980s and motivate the reader to develop, design, and implement some creative strategies to meet this change.

Elizabeth Nancy Lewis
Patricia Vince Carini

Acknowledgments

We would like to express appreciation to the enthusiastic staff of A Station, also known as the piloteers, who were fundamental in implementing total patient care and were supportive of the concepts in this book: Esther Asche, RN; Elaine Boomer, RN; Renee Casados, LVN; Alice Curtin, LVN; Leona Knoblock, NA; Cleo Oliver, LVN; Bobby Squalatti, RN; Peggy Stanwood, RN; Susan Toti, RN; and Renee Carlos Welsh, RN.

We are especially grateful to the following individuals; without their assistance in their specialized areas, writing this book would have been a most difficult process:

- Norma Anderson Badger, RN, BSW, for conceptualizing the teamsmanship approach to the participatory management model described in this book
- Elaine Boomer, RN, and Delpha Roper, RN, for the time-and-motion studies in this book
- Peggy Murray Bowe, RN, for editorial assistance with sections of the preliminary manuscript for the purpose of nursing interpretation and clarity
- Bernice Quinn, MA, MLS, for thorough help in researching our subject matter
- John P. Rinset, BS, MS, for continued support to the nursing management group at Doctors Hospital of Pinole
- Renee Carlos Welsh, RN, for assisting with typing of the preliminary manuscript and editorial assistance with a number of exhibits
- Beth Zaentz, BS, BA, MPH, CPA, for editorial assistance with the budget and reporting forms in this book

Part I

Issues in Staffing

Chapter 1

Why a Staffing System Is Needed

OBJECTIVES

Following completion of this chapter the reader will be able to:

- identify the similarities in the standards set by the American Nurses' Association (ANA) and the Joint Commission on Accreditation of Hospitals (JCAH) that pertain to nurse staffing systems,
- relate the ANA Standards of Nursing Practice and the JCAH standards to the relevancy for developing nurse staffing systems, and
- identify guidelines that should be used to develop a nurse staffing system.

Students of systems theory delight in nurse staffing systems and patient acuity systems. The Joint Commission on Accreditation of Hospitals, state licensing agencies, and the American Nurses' Association set standards for nursing care based on principles inherent in patient acuity and nurse staffing systems. On the other side of the coin nursing managers ponder them, physicians ignore them, hospital administrators and financial officers question their value for meeting profit and productivity goals, and staff nurses, who need a patient acuity system, view them as the nursing office's way of reducing staff.

One of the most critical and continuing concerns facing nursing administrators of health care delivery systems is the management and effective application of a realistic nurse staffing system based on patient acuity levels. Yet the words *nurse staffing system* or *patient acuity* often carry negative connotations to hospital and nursing administrators, physicians, and staff nurses. Most often the negative reactions of these groups is due to an incomplete understanding of how or why a staffing system can be optimally utilized to deliver comprehensive, quality nursing care and increase professional satisfaction, while justifying costs and increasing patient satisfaction.

Nursing administrators must be aware of the reasons why staff nurses often feel negative toward staffing systems in general. Staffing systems and patient acuities have somehow gained the same high level of distaste and low level of credibility as patient care plans have to the professional staff nurse. But nursing service departments need staffing systems—staffing systems that are outlined, specific, detailed, and meaningful to nursing administrators. Nursing services need staffing systems based on patient classifications or acuities. But by the same token nursing administrators need to have the responsibility and authority to create, develop, monitor, control, review, and revise those systems as often as necessary to meet the objectives and goals of the entire nursing service department.

In the same manner that the nursing department of a hospital is required to provide a written plan of care for all patients, the nursing department is required to provide and follow an established nurse staffing system and patient classification system in accordance with the JCAH requirements for hospital accreditation and with the state requirements for hospital licensure. Not only do these agencies outline what should be done—a staffing system—but wording often suggests how the system should function and what the system should reflect. Mandating a requirement often bores many creative minds in nursing administration. But before looking at the JCAH standards as another set of requirements with which to comply, one should look first at Standard II of the Standards for Nursing Service prepared by the American Nurses' Association Commission on Nursing Services. These standards are intended for use in any health care system as guidelines for nursing service.

ANA STANDARDS

ANA Standard II states, "Nursing Administration has the responsibility and authority for the quality of Nursing practice within the Health Care Organization."[1] The key words in this standard are *responsibility* and *authority*, words that are continually thrust on nursing administrators, managers, and staff nurses. "You are responsible for this patient's care," the head nurse says to the staff nurse. "The responsibility for seeing that patient care plans are complete on this unit rests with you," the nursing administrator states to the head nurse. The hospital administrator or chief financial officer looks to the nursing administrator and affirms, "You will be responsible for completing your operating budget reports by Friday at 4 P.M."

While responsibility is all around them, nursing administrators have not yet fully received the authority to follow through with these required responsibilities. More often than not, the authority given to the nursing administrator is rather vague or fragmented, if defined at all.

In some instances, although nursing administrators are given the responsibility for developing staffing patterns and staffing systems, they are not always given the authority by the hospital administrator to carry out that responsibility. Nor do they consistently receive support from the hospital administrator when the staffing system is questioned by other members of the administration, nursing staff, or medical staff.

Although ANA Standard II supports the idea that nursing administrators should have both the responsibility and authority for the quality of nursing practice, in reality the nursing administrator of the 1980s is only beginning to see the top of the management iceberg called authority, while carrying the burden of its glacier called responsibility. Along with the responsibility for the quality of nursing practice must be the authority to ensure that the quality of care be delivered in an acceptable manner.

Nursing administrations need to develop meaningful staffing systems as a step toward providing for the quality of nursing practice within the organization. Standard VIII of the ANA Standards for Nursing Service states, "Nursing Administration shall detail guidelines for utilization of nursing personnel."[2] An objective and specific nurse staffing system provides nursing administrations with tools and guidelines for adequately utilizing nursing personnel to meet this standard.

Guideline C of Standard VIII goes on to state "Nursing Administration assigns the categories of personnel to matching levels of competence in relation to consumer care needs."[3] With a well-controlled staffing system, nursing administrations can better meet this guideline by assigning nursing personnel to care for patients based on the competency level of the employee and the needs of the patient.

JCAH STANDARDS

JCAH also has set standards pertaining to staffing systems. JCAH is the accreditation commission recognized for successfully standardizing services in the health care field in the interest of improving the quality of care provided in hospitals and other health-related organizations.[4] The accreditation survey process by JCAH members is completely voluntary on the part of the hospital or organization. Although hospitals elect to participate in this accreditation survey for a number of reasons including Medicare reimbursement, the JCAH standards of quality of care and service reflect the highest state of the art in health care.

JCAH Standard III of nursing service states "Nursing department/service assignments in the provision of nursing care shall be commensurate with the qualifications of nursing personnel and shall be designed to meet the nursing care needs of the patient."[5] Although this standard seems straightforward, JCAH states in the interpretation of this standard that a number of criteria should be met to comply with this standard.

> A sufficient number of qualified registered nurses shall be on duty at all times to give patients the nursing care that requires the judgment and specialized skills of a registered nurse. Nursing personnel staffing shall also be sufficient to assure prompt recognition of any untoward changes in a patient's condition and to facilitate appropriate intervention by the nursing, medical, or hospital staffs. In striving to assure optimal achievable quality nursing care and safe patient environment, nursing personnel staffing and assignment shall be based at least on the following:
>
> - A registered nurse plans, supervises, and evaluates the nursing care of each patient;
> - To the extent possible, a registered nurse makes a patient assessment before delegating appropriate aspects of nursing care to ancillary nursing personnel;
> - The patient care assignment minimizes the risk of the transfer of infection and accidental contamination;
> - The patient care assignment is commensurate with the qualifications of each nursing staff member, the identified nursing needs of the patient, and the prescribed medical regimen;
> - Responsibility for nursing care and related duties is retained by the hospital nursing department/service when nursing students and nursing personnel from outside sources are providing care within a patient care unit.
>
> The nursing department/service shall define, implement, and maintain a system for determining patient requirements for nursing care on the basis of demonstrated patient needs, appropriate nursing intervention, and priority for care.[6]

There are a number of similarities in the standards set by the ANA commission and JCAH pertaining to nursing service and nurse staffing. The ANA commission and the JCAH standards greatly support each other's criteria. Nursing administrations should review these similarities as support and justification for providing the highest quality of care, service, and staffing.

STATE CODES

In addition to the ANA and JCAH standards that support the need for effective nurse staffing systems, nursing administrators also need to examine individual state codes pertaining to patient classifications and staffing systems in order to assure that their departments are in compliance with state requirements. For example, the California Administrative Code, Title 22, Division 5, describes the licensing and certification requirements of health facilities. Article 3, Section 70213 of California Title 22, Division 5, states:

> (e) There shall be written nursing audit procedure and evidence that audit procedures are in effect.
> (f) There shall be a method for determining staffing requirements based on assessment of patient needs. This assessment shall take into consideration at least the following:
> (1) The ability of the patient to care for himself.
> (2) His degree of illness.
> (3) Requirements for special nursing activities.
> (4) Skill level of personnel required in his care.
> (5) Placement of the patient in the nursing unit.
> (g) There shall be documentation of the methodology used in making staffing determinations. Such documentation shall be part of the records of the nursing service and be available for review.
> (h) There shall be a written staffing pattern which shall show:
> (1) Total numbers of staff, including full-time and full-time equivalents.
> (2) The available nursing care hours for each nursing unit.
> (3) The categories of staff available for patient care.
> (i) There shall be a record retained for six months of the written staffing pattern available for review by the Department at any given time.

It is most important that nursing administrations develop a coordinated staffing system that complies with individual state requirements as well as with JCAH standards and the ANA Standards for Nursing Practice. The nursing personnel needed in a nursing unit can be properly determined only by an effective system that evaluates and assesses the needs of patients concurrently with the individual capabilities of the nursing staff assigned to the unit. By the same token it is imperative that records and reports of both staffing patterns and patient acuities be consistently maintained, regularly reviewed, and revised when appropriate.

In the same way that a quality assurance program can measure the success in acquiring and meeting a standard of practice or a standard of care, a well-designed, meaningful acuity system (patient classification system) supplies the tools necessary to provide and justify adequate and appropriately skilled nursing staff to meet the standards for quality and appropriateness of nursing care.

NOTES

1. American Nurses' Association, "Standards for Nursing Services" (Kansas City, Mo.: American Nurses' Association, 1973) p. 2.

2. Ibid., p. 4.

3. Ibid.

4. Joint Commission on Accreditation of Hospitals, *Accreditation Manual for Hospitals, 1981* (Chicago: Joint Commission on Accreditation of Hospitals, 1980), p. vi.

5. Ibid., p. 117.

6. Ibid., p. 118.

Chapter 2

Turning Subservience, Servitude, and Nurturing into Quality and Accountability

OBJECTIVES

Following completion of this chapter the reader will be able to:

- describe the original nursing model and its impact on quality and accountability,
- draw correlations between the original nursing model and the current nursing educational process, and
- state the similarities between hospitals and businesses.

In the late 1960s Ralph Nader challenged the automotive industry. He said that the automobile suffered from major safety defects inherent at the time of purchase. Automotive executives protested, advocate groups cheered, and consumers struggled with a car that was unfit for safe and efficient transportation. Sometimes consumers even struggled for their lives as a result of faulty workmanship. Suddenly the emphasis shifted from the type and cost of an automobile to the quality and accountability of the manufacturer. The consumer was demanding quality and holding the automotive industry accountable for its product. *Quality* and *accountability* had become the buzzwords of the 1970s.

Quality and accountability continue to be buzzwords. Like every other industry, the health care industry has opened its ears. Quality and accountability pervade the JCAH and ANA standards for nursing care. Hospital administrators, financial analysts, nursing administrators, and staff nurses are as committed to quality patient care as Ralph Nader was to improving the automotive industry. Although the standards have been mandated, the actual process has not been specified. Nursing administrators had relied on the expertise of financial analysts to develop the process to ensure quality patient care within the confines of a budget. By developing a nurse staffing system using patient classifications, the need to rely solely on the financial analyst for the nursing department budgetary process no longer exists. Now, nursing can collect its own data to justify budgetary needs.

The evolution of staffing guidelines, patient classification systems, and patient assessment systems has been accompanied by a revolution headed by staff nurses. Mere mention of such phrases usually brings about a loud protest among nurses while any attempt at implementing patient classification systems frequently results in blatant rejection and noncompliance. A historical overview of the original nursing model will help in understanding this revolution and the subsequent dichotomy between the nursing administration and staff nurses.

ORIGINAL NURSING MODEL

The nursing model was fashioned by Florence Nightingale, a dedicated, generous, brave and rebellious person. What other woman of her time was so committed to caring and giving that she would challenge society and embark on her own adventure through swamplands and over battlefields to provide health care? Women of her time were caring and giving, but they selected the recipients, who were usually family and intimate friends.

The picture changed dramatically as a result of Florence Nightingale's endeavors. Those intrinsic characteristics of nurturing and mothering were extended beyond family and friends to include the sick, the injured, and the dying. Society created a need, and women gallantly marched to fulfill that need. Subservience and servitude, along with nurturing, became the foundation of the nursing profession—a foundation that unfortunately has not shifted significantly over the years.

Florence Nightingale's adventure did not begin and end with her travels. She not only revolutionized the entire health care system; in addition she questioned the whole issue of male supremacy by developing a structured educational system for nurses. Subsequently, the nursing profession struggled to identify itself as an autonomous profession capable of imagining, creating, thinking, defining, and implementing its own educational systems and practice.

As the nursing profession struggled for its autonomy and identity, a number of archaic philosophies toward health care began to become apparent. Following World War II the educational process not only continued to focus on both theoretical knowledge and technical skills but also attempted—and succeeded—to establish a professional group for individual patient care. That is, registered nurses (RNs), licensed vocational nurses (LVNs), nurses' aides, orderlies, and secretarial help would coordinate patient care activities according to basic theoretical knowledge learned by the RN and the routine tasks and skills mastered by LVNs, nurses' aides, orderlies, and secretarial help. The emphasis was to incorporate these workers into a group of individuals who would provide a task-oriented approach to nursing. Hence, team nursing became a reality.

A further change of these philosophies did not occur until the 1950s. More attention was devoted to assessing the efficiency of this group method of task-orientated nursing care from the standpoint of the economical use of nursing personnel. Nursing tasks, the level of care that a patient required, and the most efficient combination of staff were beginning to be considered.

Also during the 1950s came an increased awareness among hospital administrators of the relationship between delivery of quality health care and the increasing cost of providing quality care. The questions of what quality health care is and how one most efficiently and cost effectively delivers that quality became issues to be defined and considered in all phases of the hospital's operation. Nurses play a major role in delivering that cost-effective, quality patient care. As nurses sought autonomy and independence, both personally and professionally, they began to define the nursing profession according to how they defined nursing, not how others defined the profession.

In the 1960s and 1970s a still greater emphasis was placed on providing quality but individualized patient care. Cost effectiveness and cost containment ran side by side with quality and accountability; hospital and nursing administrations faced their greatest challenge.

As administrators and managers in the nursing profession, one goal is to attain a certain degree of power over the direction of the nursing profession. This is often easier said than done. As Trucia Kushner states in *Ms.* magazine, "The hospital system has exploited the nursing profession, used its cheap productivity and ignored its cravings for dignity and respect."[1]

To a certain extent this statement is accurate. However, nurses have contributed to their own exploitation by not taking a firm stand on the philosophy of the profession and demanding its recognition. This is not to endorse unionization but rather to support the idea of the nursing profession upgrading its standards of nursing education and earning its dignity and respect through its actions and performance. In other words the foundation must shift and the role of nursing must change.

THE ROLE OF NURSING EDUCATION

Thus far nursing education has steadfastly supported the nursing role of subservience, servitude, and nurturing. Entering the educational process, a nursing student usually devotes the first academic year to prerequisite courses. These courses are designed to provide the scientific knowledge needed to care appropriately for patients. By the second year, and throughout the remainder of nursing education, the student learns about the basic needs of unique patients at various times under unpredictable circumstances.

Because no one can predict the patients, the times, and the circumstances, nursing education attempts to find the common denominator, namely the basic needs of the patient. To simplify the approach, students learn that the patient has eight basic needs: safety, rest, activity, oxygen, nutrition, fluids and electrolytes, elimination, and avoidance of pain. Although students are not supposedly expected to meet all the needs, most weekly care plans would be returned as incomplete if a student chose to address only one or two needs of a patient. The conditioning process has begun. The student learns quickly that an all-encompassing, grandiose care plan must be presented every week in order to succeed. Furthermore, feelings of anxiety and guilt begin to surface if the student perceives an inability to meet all the needs of one patient. Once again, subservience, servitude, and nurturing are perpetuated through the educational process.

Upon graduation and successful completion of the tests of state licensing boards, the student is rather abruptly introduced to the extremely complex organization known as the hospital. Usually the individual is minimally prepared to cope with the day-to-day activities of hospital life. Suddenly the nurse faces the expectation of adequately caring for at least five or six patients and producing meaningful, individualized care plans. The nurse discovers that the patient is actually charged for toothpaste and toothbrush and learns that paper supplies, pens, and pencils are tightly controlled. The nurse can't understand why the hospital will purchase only plastic stethoscopes at $5 each.

The nurse shrieks, "I can't deliver quality care to my patients; we need more staff; certainly the hospital can afford to give away toothpaste; and if the hospital were really concerned about quality care, it would purchase better stethoscopes." The nurse's entire frame of reference is based on an educational experience of one patient, one care plan, and free supplies, encompassed by an undying commitment to subservience, servitude, and nurturing. Nurses find themselves holding on to that conditioning process, which will allow them to deliver the quality of care that in their minds is of utmost importance. In other words they associate the conditioning process with quality patient care. Hence, only under these circumstances will they willingly accept accountability.

SIMILARITIES BETWEEN HOSPITALS AND BUSINESSES

This frame of reference is highly unrealistic. It is this unrealistic frame of reference that tends to frustrate nurses, as well as creating friction between nursing administration and staff nurses. Roxane Spitzer observed, "It may be possible that at least some of the burnout experienced by nurses at all levels is the result of a failure to prepare nurses to function in a complex, competitive structure."[2] Nurses must become cognizant of the similarities between hospitals and other businesses. Knowledge and acceptance of these similarities may ease the shock of reality. Some similarities are:

- Hospitals may be service-oriented but they are also goal-directed and can no more afford to operate in the red than any other business.
- The hierarchical structure of hospitals is that of the traditional corporate pyramid, whereby both power and decision-making functions are delineated.
- Hospital administrators are accountable to a board of directors just as business administrators are responsible to stockholders.
- Hospitals are composed of planners, organizers, and doers.
- Performance, productivity, and management are as crucial to hospitals as they are to any other business entity.
- Hospitals are becoming more and more competitive. Just as a customer chooses a product or service, so too does the patient choose where to invest health care dollars.
- Finally, in this age of cost containment and cost effectiveness, performance, productivity, and management are dependent on the effective use of budgets.

In essence, then, a hospital *is* a business—in fact, by any measure, the largest or second largest business in the United States. Nursing is a vital component of this business. Nurses must perceive themselves as individuals who hold controlling positions within a corporate structure. This corporate structure is also an institution dependent on sound management practices in order to function. As a result nurses must be as adept in management practices and cost-benefit ratios. They must not fear management for "without institutions there is no management, but without management there is no institution."[3]

In short the original nursing model of subservience, servitude, and nurturing is ineffective. The professional arena has changed; nurses no longer function on battlefields and in swamplands but rather in complex, competitive structures. "The achievement of nurses' professional and personal goals depends on their ability to succeed in a corporate structure that is the hospital."[4] Nurses should not be held accountable for nursing care based solely on the original nursing model. Their attention should be redirected to an area, namely, the management process, where they can be assured of delivering quality patient care and willingly accept accountability.

NOTES

1. Trucia Kushner, ''The Nursing Profession—Condition: Critical,'' *Ms.*, August 1973, p. 101.
2. Roxane Spitzer, ''The Nurse in the Corporate World,'' *Supervisor Nurse,* April 1981, p. 21.
3. Ibid.
4. Ibid.

Chapter 3

The Importance of Autonomy in the Practice of Nursing

OBJECTIVES

Following completion of this chapter the reader will be able to:

- describe the factors (or forces) in the nursing environment that can cause discontent and disillusionment for the nurse and
- relate the factors in the nurse's struggle for autonomy.

Man has toiled for centuries in a competitive manner for the good of the community. He has formed organizations to maximize production from a collective effort. Automation and computer systems have relieved some of the monotony of this work. Man is far more affluent and economically independent than at any other time. Striving for this affluence and independence since the beginning of time, modern man still finds himself feeling anxious, bewildered, and empty. These feelings affect his interactions with family, friends, and fellow laborers. He is unable to cope with the family structure, his peer group, and the structure of his place of employment. In short, man is dissatisfied with those organizations that he has developed in the hopes of achieving fulfillment, enjoyment, and stability. In essence man has not experienced autonomy or self-actualization.

THE NEED FOR AUTONOMY

In many professions and careers individuals express a great need to exist in the state of autonomy. Autonomous desires pervade lives in many ways, from the goal to be independent—not only collectively as a country or a city, but also as individuals governed by independent thoughts and philosophies—to the need to experience a sense of freedom within.

Autonomy is defined by Webster as "self-government; independence."[1] Synonyms for autonomy include "freedom, liberty, scope, range, latitude, emancipation, and liberation."[2] Self-actualization, on the other hand, is an ongoing process of self-fulfillment, achieving one's mission in life, so to speak, by which one develops potential, talent, and capacity.[3] States of autonomy and the process of self-actualization, then, are unique, individual, and personal places for each person. Degrees of autonomy and self-actualization exist in differing proportions in individuals and in varying proportions at different times in life. In other words, people choose, either consciously or unconsciously, the level of autonomy, independence, self-actualization, or self-fulfillment that they wish to feel or experience internally. Likewise, an individual chooses to share with others different stages of autonomy, depending on the circumstances or factors surrounding that autonomy.

Each person exists as a unique individual in a turbulent environment. To maintain a state of equilibrium, man opposes this turbulent environment by exercising free will. To exercise free will, one must know oneself and truly be independent of the various forces that continually restrain the individual. At birth, one is totally dependent on others for survival. As one matures, instinct steers the direction toward independence (autonomy). However, the search for independence fails as the individual's preexisting standards (religious, moral, and ethical standards instilled from parental influence and formal education) dominate the thought processes. One's energies instead become directed toward rebellion. As Rollo May states:

> Since the rebel gets his sense of direction and vitality from attacking the existing standards and mores, he does not have to develop standards of his own. Rebellion acts as a substitute for the more difficult process of struggling through to one's own autonomy, to new beliefs, to the state where one can lay new foundations on which to build.[4]

Consequently the family structure with its religious, moral, and ethical standards serves as the scapegoat for man's lack of autonomy. Rather than become introspective, the individual blames parents and their beliefs for one's own vacillation and inability to make decisions, establish meaningful relationships, and maintain health. This rebellious attitude begins in early childhood and continues through adolescence and adulthood. Before long, the individual reaches adulthood from a chronological viewpoint and becomes a candidate for employment.

One's life on the job takes on projections similar to childhood and adolescent life experiences. The individual again feels frustration, ambivalence, and anger, this time toward the job and employer. Eventually the coping mechanism may manifest itself through blatant rebellion. Gradually the person rebels against the rules and regulations, dress codes, management principles, etc. This time the scapegoat is the corporation for which one works; one's unhappiness, anxiety, and bewilderment are deemed the direct result of the employer. Once again the individual shies away from developing any standards for he is too busy challenging established standards. The individual consistently blames other forces for discontent and disillusionment. In an attempt to cope, the person merely displaces all these feelings onto others.

The inability to cope with one's own feelings and actually take responsibility for oneself has impeded growth and development. The person has allowed the socialization process to paralyze natural instinct completely. The individual identifies parents and employer as the symbol of power and strength, failing to realize personal capabilities. Indeed, the process of introspection is painful, frightening, and anxiety-provoking. However, one must examine the inner conscience in order to survive in the turbulent environment. When living becomes a struggle, one cannot retreat to the familiar lifeline—the umbilical cord—nor allow the corporation to serve as a surrogate mother.

War must not be waged against society. Instead, this is an internal war against one's reluctance to seek growth, development, and health. The outcome, of course, will depend on the individual's awareness of *self*—needs, strengths, weaknesses, and beliefs. The individual must strive toward developing emotional potentials as well as physical and technical ones. Organizational life—whether it be family, peer group, or work—will benefit by one's self-awareness and consciousness. As each individual changes and becomes responsible and accountable for ideas and behavior, the family and work life will change. Once again it is not the family or work life that is truly unbearable. What is unbearable is the inability of the individuals who comprise these organizations to discover themselves—to become autonomous and enjoy self-actualization.

NURSING'S BEHAVIOR PATTERN

Does not the nursing profession in general exhibit similar behavior patterns as described by Rollo May? Nurses exist in an extremely turbulent environment—fluctuating patient acuities and daily patient census compounded by the various personalities of staff members and numerous physicians, not to mention the challenge of meeting predetermined hours per patient day, containment of supplies and operating budgets, etc. Nurses, to survive as professionals, attempt to establish a state of equilibrium within the work environment. Attempts at organizing their time and setting and reshuffling priorities in the midst of constant interruptions and uncontrollable changes in patient conditions are sometimes in vain. Staff nurses ask, "How can we establish order in an environment (hospital) that has no order? Why try?"

That a hospital has no order or that order can never be achieved in a hospital is a premise grounded in preexisting standards. Staff nurses, too, allow their formal education based on subservience, servitude, and nurturing to permeate their everyday interaction with staff and patients. As the staff nurses attempt to meet every need of every patient and fail, frustration and anger surface. They blame their inability to succeed on their education: "They (the instructors) didn't prepare us for this." Or they may blame the organization: "Nursing administration doesn't care about quality patient care."

The complaints are numerous and the resistance is blatant. Staff nurses don't have time to develop care plans, maintain acuity systems, and perform nursing assessments. Furthermore, they won't make time (by their own admission) to do any of these. It is less painful to identify the scapegoat as the university or the corporation rather than from within. The goal should be toward improvement as opposed to assigning blame. Consequently, valuable time and precious energy are wasted in criticizing and challenging the value of care plans, acuity systems, and nursing assessments. In essence staff nurses refuse to participate in such endeavors and ultimately fail to reach an autonomous state.

However, a desired level of autonomy and self-actualization is an important need, and goal, for the professional nurse. While looking at the written goals and objectives of nursing departments, one can frequently find language relevant to developing autonomy as a nursing department or demonstrating to the medical staff that nursing is an autonomous profession.

Nursing managers profess a desire to practice autonomy in nursing, to be accountable and responsible for maintaining nursing standards and for upholding the quality of nursing care they give. If these are the goals of the profession, nursing leaders must begin by exerting a perhaps latent power: the power to express what it is they need and to seek actively what they say they need.

These concepts are extremely important in laying the groundwork for any new protocol within a nursing department. It is absolutely necessary that nursing administrators be as familiar with these concepts as staff nurses are with the corporate structure. Nursing administrators must be alert to the signs and symptoms displayed by the staff nurses in their struggle for autonomy and self-actualization and must be able to convert rebellion and resistance into creativity and ingenuity. Complaints and disagreements must be heard by nursing administrators. The challenge to nursing administrators is to foster a state of autonomy by creating an environment that supports independent and individualized thinking while simultaneously keeping goals and objectives of the nursing department clearly focused in the minds of nursing managers and in conjunction with the overall goals and direction of the hospital.

NOTES

1. *The New American Webster's Dictionary*. By Andrew T. Moorhead and Philip D. Moorhead (Eds.), (New York: New American Library–Times Mirror, 1972).

2. *Roget's Thesaurus*, rev. ed. by Andrew T. Moorhead and Philip D. Moorhead (New York: New American Library–Times Mirror, 1978).

3. Marlene Grissum and Carol Spengler, *Womanpower and Health Care* (Boston: Little, Brown & Company, 1976), p. 67.

4. Rollo May, *Man's Search for Himself* (New York: Dell Publishing, Inc., 1953), p. 157.

Chapter 4

The Changing Role of the Nursing Administrator

OBJECTIVES

Following completion of this chapter the reader will be able to:

- describe how the role of the nursing administrator and the role of the physician impact one another,
- describe how the hospital administrator can impact the role of the nursing administrator,
- describe how the hospital financial controller can impact the role of the nursing administrator,
- identify the members of the hospital administrative team,
- describe the ways in which many hospital administrators are beginning to view the role of the nursing administrator as a member of the hospital administrative team,
- describe how this new image of the nursing administrator can positively impact the nursing department, and
- understand the importance of teamsmanship between the hospital administrator, the financial controller, and the nursing administrator.

THE NURSING ADMINISTRATOR AND THE MEDICAL STAFF: FRIENDS OR FOES?

Perhaps one of the key issues confronting nursing administrators is the role of the physician and the effect of this role on the nursing profession. At nearly every nursing management seminar or conference the role of the physician is discussed in reference to some nursing issue. In many cases entire seminars have been developed to educate the nursing administrator to the specific role of the physician. Surely no one would doubt that physicians, with their abundance of knowledge and wealth, permeate every facet of health care—including nursing's own continuing education programs. The response to programs highlighting the role of the physician is sometimes anything but favorable.

Primarily nurses face such a dilemma with physicians because of the role that nurses themselves have chosen to perpetuate—that of subservience, servitude, and nurturing. (The reader need only refer to Chapter 2 to gain insight into some of the reasons why this role exists.) But there is another side of the coin, namely, the role that the physician has chosen to perpetuate.

Just as the role of the nurse appears grounded in Florence Nightingale and her endeavors (Chapter 2), the role of the physician appears to be defined as early as the New Testament, where Jesus was called the Great Physician; the blind saw, the deaf heard, and the crippled walked as a result of His healing powers. Around 900 A.D. healers began to view medicine as the study of the corpse. Soon this knowledge was applied to the living body, and significant strides were made in medicine. Hippocrates left an indelible mark on medical science. It is his oath proudly stated by every medical student at graduation, an oath that has endured more than 2,000 years, as Pasteur, Lister, and Freud molded the medical profession.

Physicians either consciously or unconsciously often demonstrate an attitude of thinking of themselves as saviors and healers. Certainly their specialties and their subspecialties appear as part of their desire to be like Christ—all-knowing and all-powerful. This desire and behavior create much of the friction between physicians and nurses, although physicians and nurses are equally concerned about the welfare and care of the patient. When the surgeon's patient develops a skin rash, the dermatologist is consulted; when the internist's patient requires surgery, the cardiovascular surgeon, the thoracic surgeon, or the orthopedic surgeon is consulted; and when the surgeon's patient develops cardiac arrhythmias, the cardiologist is consulted.

The medical specialties go on and on—but not so with nursing. The surgical nurse does not refer the patient to a medical nurse when arrhythmias develop; the pediatric nurse does not consult with the medical nurse when a child develops asthma; and the medical nurse does not consult with the obstetric-gynecologic nurse when an elderly cardiac patient develops postmenopausal bleeding. Nurses are expected to manage effectively all aspects of the patient's care and naturally notify the appropriate physician in a time of need. Physicians bemoan the incompetence of the nurse while seldom realizing that as physicians specialize on one specific need of the patient, nurses are attempting to coordinate the effort between two, three, or four specialists and care for several basic needs of that same patient.

Physicians, because of their all-powerful and all-knowing attitude, believe that they can be as effective with nursing administrators as they are with their patients.

Physicians attempt to exert their awesome power on nursing administrators and feel that nursing administrators should adhere to verbal orders (''hire more staff, hire Nurse Smith, fire Nurse Jones, promote Nurse Brown, and demote Nurse Miller'') in the same manner that staff nurses adhere to their written orders.

Alert and effective nursing administrators can ill afford to follow such dictates and whims. Nursing modalities such as team nursing, total patient care, and primary nursing care concepts are beyond the physician's purview. Yet, there isn't a nursing administrator in the country who would deny that physicians attempt to direct and control nursing modalities by demanding that an individual with a certain level of training (RN versus LVN) should care for their patient or that more secretaries be hired for a unit. Perhaps not enough personnel are available at the level that the physician has requested, or the staffing pattern that the head nurse has designed for the unit does not require the use of a unit secretary for that day based on the intensity of the patient acuities. In many instances physicians have succeeded in their demands but only to the detriment of the nursing staff and the patient.

The role of the nursing administrator changed dramatically in the 1970s. Previously the head of a nursing department was looked on by the hospital administration as well as the medical staff as the chief nurse, responsible for the staffing of nursing units. This chief nurse was also expected to participate in carrying out direct hands-on clinical nursing care. Until the 1970s it was not unusual to find the chief nurse of the nursing department carrying out doctors' orders, administering injections, answering patient lights, and even serving as a member of the code team of the hospital. Because the head of the nursing department is a professional, there frequently was (and in some facilities still is) a conflict between the nurse administrator's professional and executive role internally and in the eyes of members of the medical staff and in some cases hospital administration. Often this division was seen as a way to keep the ''nurse expert'' in the clinical area and ''leave the extraneous management to other individuals with special abilities in these aspects.''[1]

THE NURSING ADMINISTRATOR AND HOSPITAL ADMINISTRATION

Until the 1980s the nursing administrator had little, if any, input into or control over the nursing department budget and administrative matters. The nursing administrator was held accountable for the outcome or bottom-line results of the department, yet the input and control were often dictated by the hospital administrator, the hospital's financial administrator (the controller), the medical staff, or all three. During the 1970s, fortunately for nurses, health care accountability changed dramatically. During this time of rising inflation and increased government subsidy of health care services, the accountability for health care delivery on the part of hospital administration, financial administration, nursing administration, and hospital medical staff became more and more an issue worthy of discussion.

The recent trend has been to view the hospital administration as a team of highly educated and specialized individuals who coordinate with one another to deliver health care to the consumer. This team includes the hospital administrator, the financial administrator, the nursing administrator, and, in many institutions, the chief of the medical staff. Thus the accountability of the administrative team of a hospital has become a greater collective issue as well as an individual challenge.

Hospital administration as a whole has been forced to deal with the quality of health care delivery and to change from individual departments of a hospital reacting to their own individual needs and concerns to a cohesive management group willing to react to the needs of other disciplines of the health care delivery system. The time has come for all departments within a hospital, including the medical staff department, to recognize their need for accountability to patient care as a team effort while at the same time establishing their credibility on an individual basis.

With this new perception of the nursing administrator as an executive member of the hospital team, hospital administrations are slowly beginning to bridge the gap between the attitudes of the past and those of the present. In many facilities the hospital administration accepts the nursing administrator as a member of this team; however, the role of the nursing administrator is still perceived in various ways, depending on the individual looking at that role. In order to solidify the role as the nurse executive of the management team, the nursing administrator needs to build collegial relationships with the executives in equivalent positions within the organization.

Unfortunately establishing a collegiality with physicians at any level does not simply happen. To build this collegiality the nursing administrator must first and foremost possess an in-depth understanding and appreciation of the traditional roles assumed by both physicians and nurses. Second, those physicians and nurses assuming traditional roles must be respected. Third, the nursing administrator must identify those physicians and nurses who view nursing and the nurse executive in a more contemporary manner. The nurse executive should not embark on an educational campaign to enlighten the traditional physician and nurse to a new concept of nursing. Instead, the nurse executive ought to focus on the process of change and educate contemporary physicians and nurses to this process.

The nursing administrator needs to exhibit through behavior and interaction with the medical staff and the nursing staff the kind of professional confidence both groups associate with effective management and administration. In this way, contemporary physicians and nurses can be called on to influence and persuade their respective peer groups over time. It is vital that the perceptions of the medical staff, nursing staff, and hospital administration regarding the nursing administrator's role be congruent.

With this long-overdue trend to identify the nursing administrator as a key part of the administrative team has been the need to identify the nurse executive as the person in charge of the nursing division of a hospital, responsible and accountable for the delivery of nursing care. The nursing administrator should be recognized as the individual responsible for the largest operating budget of the hospital and held accountable for numerous administrative matters involving decision making and quality of health care delivery within the hospital. The nursing staff expense is the largest single item in the hospital budget and comprises the most costly component of hospital operations. As the nursing department's budget increases, the role of the nursing administrator should be drawn closer to that of overall hospital administration and operations.

Although gradually receiving responsibility for this large division within the hospital, often the nursing administrator lacks access to both formal and informal power groups and is thus left in a weak position of power and authority. Issues discussed at governing board meetings frequently deal with the finances and economics of the hospital operations. When developing and maintaining control over the department's budget and expenses, the nursing administrator needs to hear firsthand the concerns of the governing board and to feel included in the distribution of those finances as well as having the responsibility, power, and authority over the nursing division.

The nursing administrator should therefore frequently attend, if not be a member of, the governing board, the long-range planning committee, the hospital's budget and finance committee, and other medical staff or hospital committees that in any way impact the nursing department or patient care. The long-range planning committee of a hospital would hardly finalize the addition of a new wing to the hospital without consulting with and including the financial controller in the planning process. Likewise, the nursing administrator, as an executive member of the hospital administrative team, should be included in any plans involving that area of expertise. Fortunately many hospitals have recognized this need and are seeking the expertise of the nursing administrator. If management authority in nursing administration is not placed in the proper perspective in the eyes of hospital administration and the medical staff, the result is a lack of control of nursing practice followed by inferior and fragmented nursing standards of patient care.

THE NURSING ADMINISTRATOR AND THE FINANCIAL CONTROLLER

Bridging the gap between nursing administration and financial administration can be one of the greatest challenges for a nursing administrator in the 1980s.

Nursing administration must employ great caution, patience, and most importantly a sense of humor in attempting to bridge this gap.

In the eyes of many nursing administrators, financial administrators (controllers) are often the most uncompromising, inflexible, and unyielding individuals employed in the health care field. Hospital financial administrators are often unable to communicate effectively with nursing administrators, either verbally or in writing, what it is they need and why they need it. The financial administrator invariably leaves piles of reports on the nursing administrator's desk to be completed within a short time. Despite vague instructions for completion often accompanying the reports, financial administrators expect the nursing administrator to know exactly how to complete these reports.

No two other individuals in a hospital organization are at further ends of the spectrum as the nursing administrator and the financial administrator. By the same token no two other individuals should be more compatible professionally than the nursing administrator and the financial administrator. In addition to their being peers as members of the hospital administrative team, the nursing administrator is responsible for the largest, most costly department of the hospital, and the financial administrator is the one key individual trained to manage and manipulate those costs and figures to the benefit of the nursing department as well as the organization.

In order to bridge this gap, nurses at all levels need to understand the different frames of reference of the nurse and the controller. The nursing administrator, through education and training as a registered nurse, has been taught dedication to patient care above all other things, a scientific approach, subjectivity, the art of assessment, and flexibility. The financial administrator, through education as a controller, does not receive an emphasis in that training to be flexible but rather to deal with hard facts. The financial administrator values exactness, specificity, and objectivity, which includes fact, figures, and budgets and leaves little room for flexibility. The contradictory fact remains: nursing administrators were not taught budget and finance in their professional education, and financial administrators were not taught differential diagnosis and disease etiology in business school.

The hospital's financial administrator for the most part has the greatest insight into the hospital's costs, expenses, and revenues. However, each hospital department head has, or ought to have, the greatest insight into how those department costs are spent and from where that revenue is generated. This insight should be from a standpoint of operational as well as capital budgets. The concerned financial administrator recognizes the expertise of each department head and utilizes these individuals within the hospital as resources for assuring greater accuracy in the budgetary process. The alert financial administrator recognizes the importance of including department heads in the budgetary process and assumes some responsibility for teaching this process to department heads, realizing that other department heads may not be familiar with the financial operations of the hospital. The financial administrator, while wanting to develop an accurate budget, should seek input from all department heads to prevent unnecessary costs and spending and reduce the possibility of purchasing antiquated or outdated capital equipment. At the same time, the sharing of expertise between the department head and the financial administrator may help the department head to understand why contracting with a particular outside service may not be as financially sound as the department head thought.

As shown in Exhibit 4-1, the changing role of the nursing administrator presents great challenges for the nursing administrator of the 1980s, who must be able to "explain to non-nurse administrators differences in levels of nursing care and relate those differences to a price tag."[2] The nursing administrator must learn how to speak the language of the hospital administrator and financial controller. An

---

Exhibit 4-1 The Plight of the Nursing Administrator

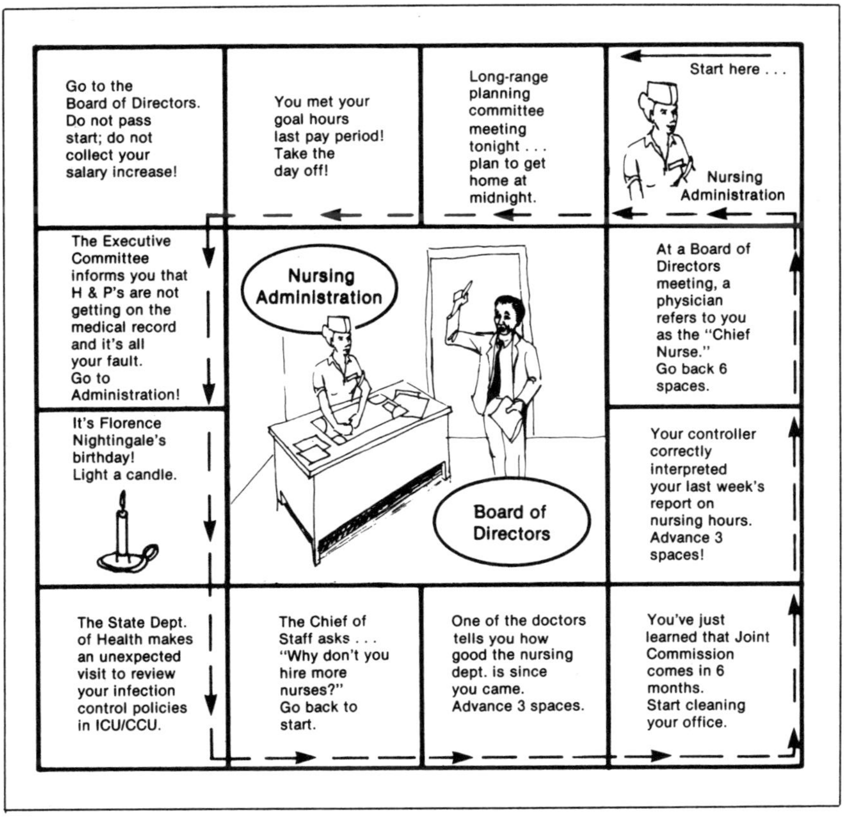

additional responsibility and great challenge is educating the hospital administrator and financial controller "to the language and significance of nursing."[3]

The hospital management team consists of the hospital administrator, the financial administrator, and the nursing administrator. There ought not be a limitation in the communication between members of this team; however, on occasion the needs and goals of these individuals may vary. It is of vital importance that each member of the management team define differences and develop an understanding of each other's area of expertise. Each department's performance is dependent on this understanding and impacts the common goals and objectives of the hospital proportionately.

NOTES

1. Barbara J. Stevens, *The Nurse as Executive* (Wakefield, Mass.: Nursing Resources, 1980), p. 88.
2. Ibid., p. 89.
3. Ibid.

Chapter 5

The Process of Change as It Relates to the Professional Nurse

OBJECTIVES

Following completion of this chapter the reader will be able to:

- state the conditions that must exist to implement successful change and
- compare and contrast the methods of change.

Another important issue that must be addressed is change. Life is in constant motion. Society has always had to cope with this movement and therefore with change to some extent. But change is occurring so rapidly that both people and organizations are distressed by it. In fact, people and organizations are so distressed by change that they attempt to suppress it. Modern technology has indeed increased the human life span, but it has done nothing to increase one's tolerance for change. Rather than suppress change and attempt to remain static in a turbulent environment, people must learn how to manage change. And "the management of change like the management of anything else, requires skill and talent."[1] To survive in this era of change, people must begin to view change management as an integral part of the management process; "change has become too important to leave to chance."[2]

CONDITIONS NECESSARY FOR CHANGE

Successful change follows a specific pattern of events. In order to implement successful change, certain conditions must exist. Too often lack of such knowledge has resulted in substantial waste in time, money, and resources. What may have been a good method to bring about change, in actuality may have caused no change at all, only a temporary change, or change accompanied by many unplanned and undesirable consequences. The study of change has done much to pave the way for productive change.

First and foremost, people must feel pressure—both internal and external—in order to be ready for change. For administrators, high rates of turnover or absenteeism, high grievance rates, and complaints and hostility can create internal pressures that will bring about change. External pressures such as the government—both state and federal—physicians, and unions can effect change within a hospital. Internal pressures that result in poor productivity, thereby jeopardizing patient care, may precipitate external pressure in the name of competition. Once a facility acquires a poor reputation, its competitive drive decreases. Such pressures tend to result in changes in leaders or leadership behavior. These same pressures also cause reexamination of practices and problems.

Second, the base of participation in change must be broadened. Instead of limiting the responsibility for change to an elite class, it should be popularized. Participation and involvement of people in defining the problems and reexamining practices are needed to build the commitment essential to effect change. A collaborative effort not only will assure higher quality solutions to problems but also will assure that behaviors and attitudes once changed remain changed.

Third, new ideas, models, or concepts must be brought in from the outside to help individuals discover new and different management practices. Employees must have access to alternative management styles.

Fourth, innovations must be limited in scope. Change should not be introduced throughout an entire organization until its feasibility and practicality have been demonstrated and learning has occurred from small-scale experimentation or a pilot program.

Fifth, a skilled leader or consultant is often necessary to develop new ideas, continue the process of reexamination, and support people as they move through change.

METHODS OF CHANGE

Basically three methods may be employed to bring about change. Two of these methods—evolutionary and revolutionary—are as old as history. The third method, systematic development, is a rather new and innovative approach to change.

The evolutionary method of change attempts to face and solve each problem as it arises, day by day, situation by situation. Consequently change is generally small and performed in a piecemeal fashion. The boundaries of the status quo remain intact while traditions and customary practices are unchallenged. Because these evolutionary modifications fit well within the boundaries of the status quo, they seldom generate authentic enthusiasm, deep resistance, or dramatic results.

To advocates of the status quo, any change represents forward progress—forward progress that is easily understood, readily accepted, and painstakingly slow.

However, evolutionary modifications and adjustments can prevent significant change. Problems that surface may be only superficial in nature while the deeper and more significant problems are unnoticed. The mere fact that a do-not-trespass sign on the boundaries of the status quo is strictly enforced may be a real barrier to progress. Prevailing values and deep-seated traditions often constitute rigidities that prevent problems from being accurately identified.

In contrast the revolutionary method of change is anything but accepting of the status quo and its assumptions and practices. Generally, revolutionary change is employed when the situation is so intolerable that evolutionary modifications are viewed as insufficient. Those traditional assumptions and customary practices embedded in evolutionary change are overthrown by revolutionary change. Revolutionary change demands acceptance of new ideas and new expectations, most likely by exercising power and authority to assure compliance—and rapidly.

Although more risks are involved in revolutionary change, the outcome is often better than either remaining in neutral gear or pursuing an evolutionary course. The change may bring about dramatic results, which may be either positive or negative. From a positive viewpoint deep-seated and long-standing problems may be fundamentally solved. Underlying tensions and anxieties may come to the forefront and be channeled into positive productivity. On the other hand, underground resistance, blatant resentment, and sabotage are common negative results.

Both the evolutionary and revolutionary approaches are highly characteristic of American corporate life. Both approaches have enjoyed their share of success. This, however, does not mean that they remain sound approaches to change.

Systematic development is a new, scientific way to manage change. Its focus is neither acceptance nor rejection of the status quo; rather, it focuses on an intellectual model of the ideal or what should be. The characteristics of the model are based on theory, logic, and fact. The model is pretested against possible circumstances over a definite period. This model will specify clear-cut objectives and results within a certain time frame. Hence, the model becomes a blueprint of what should be and not of what is.

It is of utmost importance that the model represent the ideal as opposed to the idealistic. Unlike ideal thinking, which is objective in nature and based on theory, logic, or fact, idealistic thinking tends to be subjective in nature and based on assumptions embedded in the status quo of what is wanted or what is desired. These wants and desires, because of personal biases, will not withstand theoretical, logical, and factual testing. This is not to say that the status quo should be taken for granted or ignored. On the contrary it is absolutely necessary that the status quo be studied in order to determine what it should be. In this way, strengths and weaknesses can be identified and compared to the ideal model. This comparison promotes objectivity and motivation among individuals. Rationalization, self-deceptions, and ingrained habits of the status quo no longer obscure the total picture of the situation.

Once the discrepancies between the actual and the ideal have been identified, planned and programmed change is possible. These discrepancies create tension and anxiety among people. As a result people begin to focus their attention on a viable solution to the problem. Their energy is channeled toward the orderly production of change, whereby steps of development are planned and programmed for implementation. Enthusiastic support ensues, not underground resistance. Individuals become involved in the organization and committed to its objectives. Their capacity to reason and analyze problems increases dramatically; risk and failure are minimal because the changes have been pretested before implementation.

In summary, both evolutionary and revolutionary changes take place naturally. Their place in history is just that—history. Systematic development, on the other hand, parallels scientific methods used to design experiments and verify results. It is a viable method to introduce change in this scientific age. Although the method may be unknown to nurses, the process is not. Nurses at all levels must begin to apply their knowledge of the scientific method to their everyday work environment.

NOTES

1. Lee Grossman, *The Change Agent* (New York: Amacom, 1974), p. 11.
2. Ibid.

Chapter 6

Management Principles To Bring about Desired Change

OBJECTIVES

Following completion of this chapter the reader will be able to:

- identify how meaningful change can positively affect patient care,
- identify how meaningful change can positively affect hospital staff, and
- identify how meaningful change can positively affect the nursing department budget.

Principles of sound management are ubiquitous; the same principles that apply to management of a nursing department apply to management of a battleship. The difference is not in what one manages but how one manages. Developing sound management philosophies with sound management principles brings about the desired results.

Sound management principles include an unselfish philosophy and an attitude of extension to others. John F. Kennedy's famous quotation not only applies to a giving attitude toward a country but also can apply to sound management philosophies and mature management attitudes: "Ask not what good management will do for me, but what I can do to be a good manager." The successful managers are concerned with the outcome of management style in terms of patient care and quality and staff satisfaction and not with how management style makes them look.

When the nursing department has decided to research alternative methods of patient classification systems used for nurse staffing, nursing managers need to be familiar with three aspects of change:

1. How will this change affect the patients?
2. How will this change affect the nursing staff?
3. How will this change affect the budget?

HOW WILL THIS CHANGE AFFECT THE PATIENTS?

When a nursing department selects a patient classification system or staffing system or makes any significant change, a most important point to consider is how the system or the change from a previous system will affect patient care. One should also ask, In what ways will the outcome of patient care or the quality of care be affected, if at all? Of paramount importance is the outcome the change creates. Is it a positive or negative outcome? What effect, if any, will the change to a new system have on patient care?

Many nursing departments have at one time or another used a subjective patient classification system, one that relied on little patient assessment by a member of the nursing staff. As a result, daily nursing care plans, if completed at all, were kept neither current nor specific to meet the changing needs of the patient as that person progressed through the hospital stay. Often the end result was inadequate communication between nursing personnel regarding the patient's needs; thus fragmented care was the outcome.

If the same nursing department chooses to change to a more objective patient classification system, one that requires the nurse actually to look at the patient, review the patient's medical record, and complete a comprehensive patient assessment both on admission and on a predetermined regular basis—i.e., every 24 hours or every shift—the end result seems obvious. Nursing care plans can be completed accurately and timely, communication between care givers improves through the patient classification system being kept up to date, and one would expect a favorable effect on patient care, at least from a nursing standpoint.

HOW WILL THIS CHANGE AFFECT THE NURSING STAFF?

Developing a change in a patient classification system and staffing system will affect the nursing staff because they are the individuals using the new system. Including members of the nursing staff in the development of the system aids in affecting the staff in a positive way. But the word *staff* should be thought of in a much broader sense. Nursing departments should also consider what effect the change to a new system may have on the staff in other hospital departments. Will ancillary department staff be affected in any way by the new system? Will the new system mean a revision of the care plan to include input from physical therapy, pharmacy, and dietary and social services on the patient's written care plan? In the state of California an interdisciplinary approach to the patient's plan of care is a requirement. The California Administrative Code, Title 22, Division 5, Article 3, Section 70213-d, states:

> (d) There shall be a written patient care plan developed for each patient in coordination with the total health team. The plan shall include

goals, problems/needs and approach and shall be available to all members of the health team.

As a result, How will this change affect the staff? becomes an extremely important question to ask because the impact of a new patient classification system means an interdisciplinary approach to the patient care plan involving a number of departments along with nursing.

Dealing with this in a positive way should include the department head in the planning and implementation stages of the new system. Sound management means communicating with and including all individuals who could be concerned with the issues involved in the new system.

Nursing departments should go one step further by asking, Will the new system in any way affect the medical staff, and if so, in what ways? The importance of footwork and politicking with the medical staff cannot be overemphasized to ensure the desired results and prevent possible disastrous results if the medical staff is not properly informed on issues that in any way affect or relate to the medical community or to patient care delivery.

HOW WILL THIS CHANGE AFFECT THE NURSING DEPARTMENT'S BUDGET?

Cost containment, cost effectiveness, and budgetary demands are constant concerns for nursing administrators. With rising inflation and fluctuating government financing of health care services, the accountability to control costs within all departments of a hospital becomes an essential challenge. The public's expectation of a health care facility is to provide the patient and the community with the highest quality of health care. On the other hand, the government's expectation is quality care within specific and defined boundaries. The accountability for the cost as well as the quality of care rests in the hospital system.

Staffing a hospital with nursing personnel is the largest single item in the hospital budget. In many hospitals over 50 percent of the employees work in the nursing department, and therefore over 50 percent of the salaries, wages, and benefits (SWBs) are absorbed by the nursing department. Yet, while the nursing department comprises the most costly aspect of hospital operations, the question of staffing patient care units is frequently one of the most obvious and quickly sought out focuses for cost containment controls.

The need for a cost containment program in the nursing department is one of the most difficult concepts to impress on all levels of nursing personnel from supervisors to staff nurses. During academic nursing programs, student nurses do not receive education, nor gain insight, pertaining to the need for budgetary concerns in a hospital setting. Because of this lack of familiarity with the budget process, nursing personnel often have a difficulty in accepting the need to contain costs. The academic training of nurses emphasizes the care of the patient; attaching a dollar sign to that care somehow leaves a bitter feeling with the concerned, committed nurse.

The dichotomy continues: government regulations on the one hand demanding explicit cost accountability on the part of hospitals for services, while on the other hand the patient and the public demanding the accountability of the hospital for the quality of care. Any decisions that result in a change of nurse staffing can have a direct impact on the cost of health care delivery and the quality of patient care and must be implemented with great caution. An adequate number of nurses can be budgeted for a given period; however, even with the best staffing plan, problems can and do occur. As the census goes up and nurses work harder, absenteeism can increase, thus resulting in paid unproductive hours or hours paid to sick time rather than to actual hours worked. "Hospitals pay a stiff price for absenteeism and turnover, including overtime pay, cost of replacement personnel, and productivity losses."[1] As the census rises and nurses work harder, nursing turnover and burnout become other problems, resulting in as high as 70 percent annual turnover in some nursing departments."[2]

Staff nursing personnel often have difficulty understanding the rationale behind the need for a nursing department to maintain a rigid budget and cost containment programs. Therefore, nursing administrations must impress on those individuals responsible for developing the new system that any change of the system that results in a change or an increase in cost must be looked at carefully and critically. When devising a new classification system or staffing system, nursing departments must look at their current costs and evaluate the effect of a change on these costs. If a change to a new system results in increased cost but can show measurably a more desirable quality of paticnt care, the nursing administration must be able to present to the hospital administrator and financial controller appropriate justification for changing to the new system.

NOTES

1. R. Bell, "Diagnosing Nursing Costs," *Cost Containment Newsletter* 22, no. 10: 3 (October 1982).
2. Ibid.

Chapter 7

Decentralization of Nursing Functions: An Essential Process for Creative Nurse Staffing

OBJECTIVES

Following completion of this chapter the reader will be able to:

- identify the advantages for a nursing department to decentralize,
- list five qualities necessary for decentralization in a nursing department,
- list four favorable outcomes of decentralizing a nursing department,
- describe the difference between performance accountability and service accountability,
- describe the objectives of a nursing administrative committee,
- list the individuals who comprise the nursing administrative committee,
- list the functions of the nursing administrative committee,
- describe the rules for effective decentralization, and
- describe how decentralization of a nursing department is essential for making a staffing system work.

Nursing has traditionally been organized along lines of autocratic authority with little room for input at the management level. Nursing directors (nursing administrators) were characterized as being as flexible as Attila the Hun and as open to the doctrine of shared power as Marie Antoinette. However, since the 1970s nursing administrators have been changing and most have accepted innovation in their authority with positive results.[1] Nursing leaders must develop an organizational structure and process that promote participatory management as opposed to autocratic management.

Decentralization of control and decision making is one way to promote autonomy in a nursing department. Decentralization is an essential process in order for a staffing system based on patient acuities to function properly and cost effectively.

The result of decentralization can be a more open philosophy among nursing leaders and elimination of the frequent unrest in the traditional hospital structure, where power, authority, and accountability were centered at the top of the nursing department.[2] If nursing administrators can learn to share power and authority with middle managers while at the same time identifying with their own levels of responsibilities, nursing departments will progress.

Decentralization is a method of structured organization where the power and the authority for decision making and change exist with the individuals most closely concerned with the decision or the change. Decentralization is also an essential element for creating a meaningful and workable staffing system. By creating open lines of communication between nursing managers, a more comprehensive staffing system can result.

QUALITIES NEEDED TO DECENTRALIZE A NURSING DEPARTMENT

For decentralization to develop in a nursing department, a number of qualities must exist.

A Desire to Decentralize

There must be an enthusiastic desire on the part of nursing managers to decentralize. Decentralization can be a major step for the development of autonomy for the professional nurse employed within the system. Nursing managers need to understand the definition of decentralized nursing management and relate this definition to how it will affect their role and increase their power and authority for decision making and change. Since decentralization brings about increased decision making at the unit level, nursing managers need to feel comfortable in making independent decisions.

Goals and Objectives Defined

Unit coordinators (head nurses) and supervisors must clearly define the goals and objectives of their unit to their unit staff. This must be done in a timely and appropriate manner to enable acceptance of the goals by each nursing staff member of the unit. Objectives of the nursing unit should be specific, measurable, and unambiguous. Goals and objectives of each unit should be in writing, should be congruent with the goals and objectives of the nursing department, and should include the method of process to be followed in order to meet the desired goals of both the unit and the nursing department. As with the development of a patient classification system (patient acuity system), the development of goals and objectives of a nursing unit should include all members of that unit.

Leadership

There must be strong leadership abilities in the key management individuals, i.e., the head nurses, unit coordinators, and supervisors in the nursing department. The nursing administration must look clearly at the mix of the staff in each unit as well as the capabilities of the members of the staff when selecting the unit coordinator (head nurse) or supervisor of that unit. Individuals respond differently to different leadership styles. Different styles of leadership are appropriate for different management settings.

Openness

An openness and a feeling of trust must exist between all members of the nursing administrative team, and there must be open lines of communication among all members. Because individual personalities of members of the nursing administrative team can and do often become a basis of conflict, any issues pertaining to change or power in authority struggles can become emotional. Whenever change takes place, individuals tend to feel insecure. Nursing administrators need to develop a one-on-one trust with the nursing middle managers (supervisors and unit coordinators) and demonstrate this trust by backing the managers when their own staff may question any change or may even question or challenge the managers themselves.

Guidance by Nursing Administration

Nursing administration must give guidance and direction in order to develop a unified organization rather than a disjointed department. Nursing administrators should hold regular, scheduled, informal meetings with individual members of the middle management team as well as group meetings. Nursing administrators need to communicate to the nursing middle managers their own understanding of decentralization concepts and also their expectations of the decentralization process. As the role of the nursing middle managers expands and their responsibility increases, so do the nursing administrators' role change and responsibilities increase. Nursing middle managers need to feel that they still have the support and the ear of nursing administration in order to prevent feelings of abandonment.

The results or positive outcomes of decentralizing a nursing department include but are not limited to:

- An increase in acceptance of accountability on the part of the nursing managers. Nursing managers through decentralization of a department can justify nursing hours and can justify an increase or decrease in nursing hours, overtime hours, and acuity levels.

- Increased unit control for the quality of patient care.
- Increased decision making in a realistic, timely manner.
- Increased respect felt from hospital administration and the medical staff as nursing managers demonstrate their ability and competence to make sound professional management decisions.

Through decentralization of nursing functions, nursing managers are more aware of the ramifications of their performance as managers and the attention that they give to their subordinates' ideas and input regarding the management of the nursing unit. The unit manager becomes more responsible for the appropriateness of the unit's scheduled staff hours, the frequency of overtime, and the accuracy of daily patient acuity reporting. The more accurate and thorough the communication, the better the patient acuity system should function.

Nursing decentralization is not a unique concept. If implemented carefully, it can be of great satisfaction to nursing administration. Nearly any nursing department in any hospital can decentralize. Yet decentralizing a nursing department is not easy. Creating change is always a difficult process. A number of principles have been identified for effective decentralization of a nursing department—rules that need to be reviewed with the members of the nursing administrative team and followed by all members of nursing administration. Exhibit 7-1 shows 12 principles for effective decentralization.

Decentralization of the nursing function encourages participation in the group process, gives ownership to problems as well as issues of a positive nature, promotes a feeling of commitment, and is essential to professional pride and professional growth. Through decentralization, the control for staffing a nursing unit and the control for monitoring the patient acuity system of a nursing unit become the responsibility and authority of the unit coordinator (head nurse). Giving this kind of control to unit coordinators increases their accountability and results in increased communication between the unit coordinator and the nursing staff; more comprehensive patient care plans; a decrease in incidents, patient complaints, and procedural errors; and thus improved patient care.

DEFINING THE ORGANIZATIONAL STRUCTURE OF THE NURSING DEPARTMENT

It cannot be overemphasized that the nursing administration needs to define the organizational structure of the nursing department. As decentralization of the nursing function occurs, members of the nursing administrative group need to understand their role and how it relates to the roles of others in the group.

Figure 7-1 is an example of a traditional organizational chart. With this style of an organizational chart, nursing administrations feel that this traditional organiza-

Exhibit 7-1 12 Rules for Effective Decentralization

D o get to know each other! Learn what your peers are all about. You'll find you have more in common than you imagined.

E xplain what you need! Most of us can not read minds . . . we have to tell people what we need. Give plenty of time to good explanation.

C ommunicate! Communicate! Communicate! . . . Not behind each other's back but face to face. Lack of communication or inadequate communication only breeds frustration. Remember, communication needs to be horizontal as well as vertical.

E xercise your expertise! You are an expert in your area. Use the skills and knowledge you have to meet your unit's goals. And don't forget about the other guy!!! He or she may benefit from your knowledge. Don't be afraid to give it away!

N ever pass the buck! Don't say, "That's not my problem" or "That's not my unit," for soon it may well become your problem. Help your peers solve problems; you'll probably learn something new.

T ogetherness is part of decentralization too! Back each other. A feeling of esprit de corps is the fundamental key to effective decentralization.

R espect each other's territory! Don't go off on a power struggle of your own. Decentralization allows plenty of power and space for all!

A sk for help! You have a lot of answers, but don't fool yourself into thinking you have all the answers. Seek out other experts in the group. Ask for help and be grateful you can learn new ideas.

L isten to each other! And listen to yourself! Try to look at the problem through the other person's eyes. Pay attention to detail. What may be your peer's problem today could be your frustration tomorrow.

I deas should be shared! When one of your peers is having a problem, don't wait to be asked, offer your great creative ideas. Do more than you have to to help others. Good ideas, like knowledge, are meant to be shared.

Z oom in on problems when they occur! Stewing over problems only makes matters worse and people angry. Hit your problems head on . . . but remember to be diplomatic!

E xpect positive results! Murphy's law of why things go wrong has no place in decentralization. Expect positive outcomes, knowing anything that *can* work, *will* work, providing we work on it together!

tional model merely shows performance accountability; that is, this chart shows which individuals report to whom and which individuals have responsibility for other members of the department, such as LVNs, nurses' aides, and ward clerks. Although it is necessary to show performance accountability and it is a fact of nursing administration that people report to other people, the traditional model separates individuals of the group by the clearly spelled-out supervisor-subordinate relationship, as shown in Figure 7-1. In an attempt to develop a participatory management style, the authors wanted to show that performance accountability can be looked at in a circular model, which shows how all individuals of the nursing management team interface with one another, placing less emphasis on the supervisor-subordinate relationship but rather bringing individuals of the group together through a team approach with a central goal.

Figure 7-2 is an example of a decentralized organizational chart showing performance accountability. This chart still reflects who reports to whom but shows better how the support or resource staff—inservice education/staff development, nurse recruiter, admissions coordinator, social services, utilization review, discharge planner, and infection control coordinator—act as a resource staff for the line positions—assistant administrator of nursing services, director of nursing, assistant directors, supervisors, and unit coordinators.

With decentralized nursing, from the standpoint of performance accountability, all unit operations, including staffing, become the responsibility of the unit coordinator or unit supervisor. Likewise, unit coordinators and unit supervisors are held accountable for unit operations.

Whenever possible, staffing and decisions for allocation of personnel should be done at the unit level. However, this cannot always occur due to the 24-hour operation of the hospital and the eight-hour shift of the unit coordinator or the unit supervisor.

Unit coordinators or unit supervisors should complete the six-week schedules for their units as described by contract agreements, if the facility has contract agreements. After completion of the six-week schedule and before posting that schedule, the unit coordinators and supervisors should submit to each assistant director of nursing their schedules for the assistant director's review. This should be done collectively, with all assistant directors, unit coordinators, and supervisors present, and should be completed the week before posting the schedule.

Through performance accountability charts one can define the ownership of tasks and responsibilities, i.e., who completes work schedules and who has responsibility for the proper functioning of the nursing unit. In addition to performance accountability, there exists in a nursing department (and in an entire hospital) an additional accountability, service accountability. Through service accountability it can be shown how individuals interface with one another to provide a service—in this case, patient care.

Figure 7-1 Traditional Organizational Chart Showing Performance Accountability

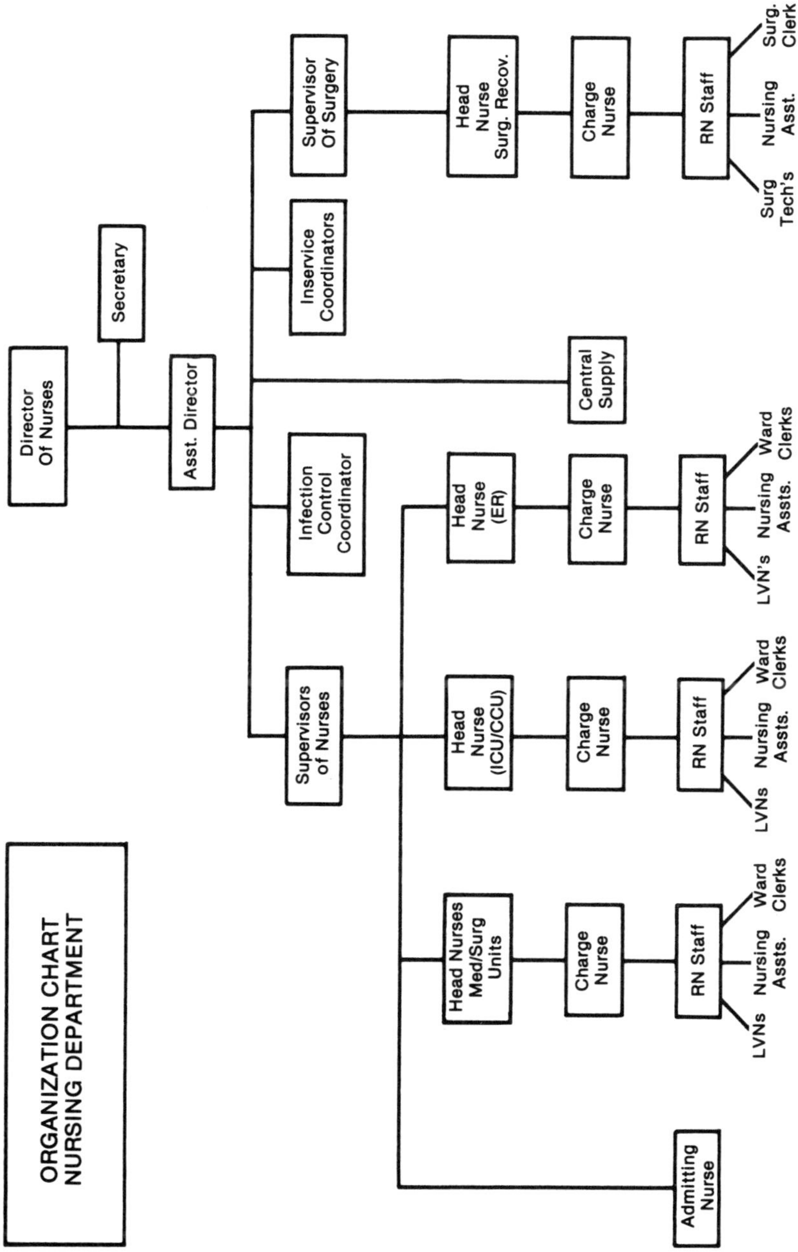

Figure 7-2 Organizational Chart Showing Performance Accountability

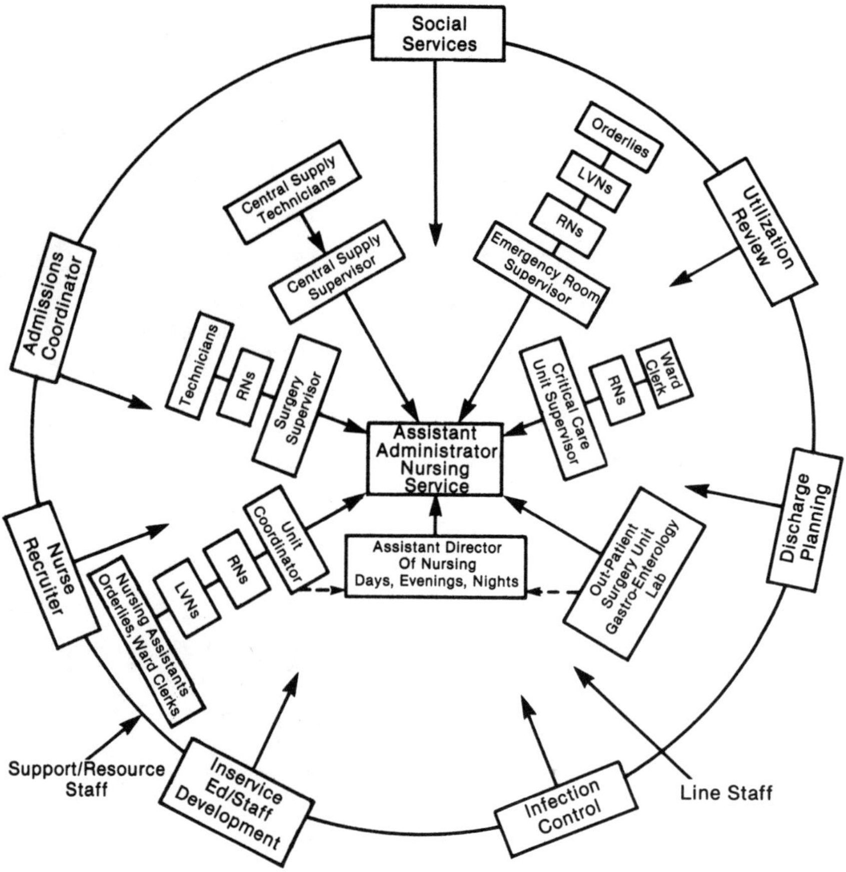

Figure 7-3 is an example of an organizational chart showing service accountability, with the patient in the center of the chart to signify the patient as the recipient of the service. In this chart, all hospital departments and services are represented. Patient care/nursing care staff refers to all departments of the hospital that provide a direct service to the patient. This includes radiology, physical therapy, dietary, central service, cardiology, pharmacy, and even the business office services and the purchasing departments because they too provide a service to the patient.

Figure 7-3 Organizational Chart Showing Service Accountability

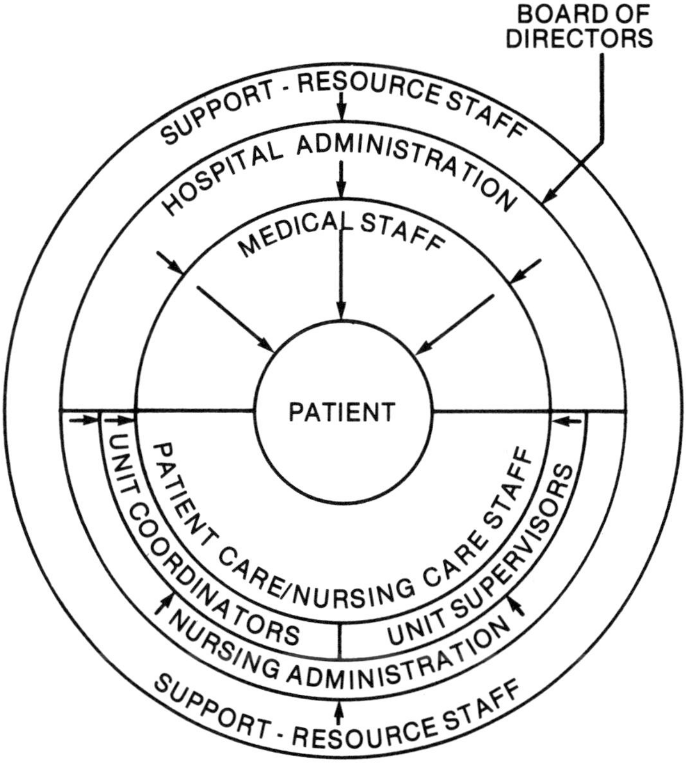

In addition to the standard organizational chart that shows performance accountability, the purpose of a chart showing service accountability is to differentiate two levels of accountability in the health care field. One level, performance accountability, describes who is responsible for which task and to which supervisor. The second level, service accountability, describes how all functions of the hospital exist to service the primary reason for the hospital's existence, that of providing service to the patient, the health care consumer. These charts are included in a discussion of decentralization of function because both performance accountability and service accountability assert that individual members of a department as well as the departments themselves are accountable and responsible for tasks as well as for patient care.

NURSING DEPARTMENT ADMINISTRATIVE COMMITTEE: A METHOD TO DEVELOP PARTICIPATORY MANAGEMENT

The advantages of collaboration and pride that come with decentralized nursing are most apparent through the nursing administrative committee. A nursing administrative committee can be developed in any nursing organization. At the authors' hospital the nursing administrative committee meets one working day per month and is dedicated to the sharing of information and problem solving among the nursing management group. Attendance can be open to all nursing managers within the hospital and can be tailored by the nursing administrator to fit the department's needs.

Frequently guest speakers may be asked to attend and address an issue that pertains to their department and nursing. Guest speakers might include the directors of public relations, financial services, physical therapy, and hospital administration. The financial administrator may be asked to present the capital and operational budget process for the next fiscal year. Participation in nursing administrative day builds further experience in the group communication process, and rapport is built with one another.

Creating a nursing department administrative committee is a method to develop the nursing department into a resource team. This resource team, by its own initiative, creates a style of participatory management and essentially decentralizes itself. In order for both decentralization and participatory management to be successful, certain qualities must be present before implementing decentralized nursing, namely:

- a desire to decentralize on the part of the nursing middle managers
- defined goals and objectives of decentralizing
- strong leadership abilities in the middle managers
- openness and trust between members of the nursing administration
- guidance and direction by the nursing administration to the middle managers

Objectives of the Nursing Administrative Committee

Using a scientific problem-solving approach, the nursing administrative committee:

- discusses existing practices in the nursing departments,
- identifies deficiencies in the system of nursing care,
- develops methods to correct deficiencies in quality,
- implements improvements through systematic analysis and planning,

- makes recommendations to the appropriate unit or department for changes or corrections in deficiencies,
- annually reviews and updates all nursing policies and procedures as indicated by current standards,
- writes standardized nursing procedures as necessary, and
- takes action on issues that will affect the nursing process.

Composition of the Nursing Administrative Committee

The nursing administrative committee consists of two groups of nursing managers. Group 1 includes the nursing administrator, assistant directors of nursing, emergency department supervisor, critical care supervisor, operating room supervisor, unit coordinators, inservice education directors, infection control coordinator, central service supervisor, utilization review and discharge planner, and nurse recruiter. Group 2 includes the relief nursing supervisors, patient admissions coordinator, and shift charge nurses. Attendance is required of individuals in group 1 and is encouraged of individuals in group 2.

All sectors of nursing are requested to serve periodically on ad hoc committees designed to accomplish the preceding objectives. Staff nurses may be asked to serve on appropriate ad hoc committees; their inclusion can be an important asset toward accomplishing the task of the ad hoc committee. The staff nurses may be more directly involved with the policy or procedure discussed at the ad hoc committee level; including them in the change process aids to develop a teamsmanship attitude and can demonstrate once again that people support what they help create.[3] Representatives from other departments may also be requested to aid by serving on appropriate ad hoc committees for solving intradepartmental problems or clarifying issues.

The chairperson of the nursing administrative committee is the nursing administrator or a designate, who would probably be one of the assistant directors of nursing.

Functions of the Nursing Administrative Committee

The nursing administrative committee discusses projects and plans, interprets state or JCAH requirements for nursing, and develops solutions, examining the potential effect of the solution or decision on patient care. Considerations are made for cost effectiveness, work productivity, and motivational aspects that can lead to job satisfaction. Through small working groups, projects and methods of improvement are presented the following month to the entire nursing administrative committee for further discussion and final approval by the committee. The committee may provide necessary feedback of information to allow for further improvements of the project. The committee as a whole critiques all projects, plans, policies, and procedures and approves or amends them.

The individuals selected for the ad hoc committees are determined by the nature of the problem, project, policy, or procedure; individuals may volunteer or be appointed to serve on an ad hoc committee. This can allow all members of the administrative committee to work on a variety of projects in the department with peers who bring a different focus to the group. Time frames are assigned to each working group project; this provides for project deadlines.

Nursing Administrative Committee Meetings

The nursing administrative committee meets monthly for one full day. Attendance at all meetings is documented in the recorded minutes and kept on file in the nursing administrative offices. A written request by a member of group 1 to be excused from a committee meeting for vacation, etc., must be submitted to the nursing administrator one week before the committee meeting. The minutes of all meetings are recorded and are available to all members of the nursing administrative committee.

Throughout nursing administrative day, all members of the group learn from one another through the exchange of information. Individuals become resources to one another; this has a great impact on increasing the sense of cohesiveness of the individuals who comprise the nursing administrative committee. Thus meaningful change takes place through the teamsmanship displayed by the members of the group, and a sense of comradery and pride exist as being part of the team.

NOTES

1. Norma Badger, coordinator of utilization review, discharge planning and social services, Doctors Hospital, Pinole, California. From speech entitled: "The Patient Resource Team," Association of Western Hospitals Convention. San Francisco, April, 1982.

2. Joan Nietz Althaus et al., *Nursing Decentralization: The El Camino Experience* (Rockville, Md.: Aspen Systems Corporation, 1981), p. 1.

3. Norma Badger.

Part II

Developing, Implementing, and Evaluating a Staffing System

Chapter 8

Examining Patient Classification Systems

OBJECTIVES

Following completion of this chapter the reader will be able to:

- define a patient classification system,
- list the three basic styles of patient classification systems, and
- list advantages and disadvantages of each style.

Nurse staffing based on a patient classification system is only one aspect of staffing, yet it is the foundation for the staffing aspect of a nursing department. A classification system must be reliable, objective, flexible, and easily interpretable. Developing a well-thought-out, realistic patient classification system is the first step toward sound staffing.

The use of a patient classification system according to nursing care requirements has become a widely accepted method of determining realistic nurse staffing patterns. Yet developing a patient classification system is a tiring and trying task. Nevertheless, a nurse staffing system that is based on patient classifications, is developed with care, and utilizes the staff nurses' input into the system can be an effective way to recruit and retain nursing staff.

A patient classification system, or patient acuity system, can be defined as the systematic identification and assessment of the individualized nursing care requirements of a group of patients. Nursing departments have developed patient classification systems in response to a great variety of needs, including documented requirements from state nurses' associations, accepted codes and practices, and the great fluctuation in the complexity of nursing care that a patient may require on a day-to-day or even a shift-to-shift basis. As nursing administrations are aware, the actual number of patients on a nursing unit is not an accurate barometer of the complex variations in nursing care that may be required by those patients. Developing a system that reflects to some degree an accurate level or extent of measurable nursing care required is an appropriate and realistic way to project nursing resources needed to provide the optimal level of nursing care mandated and desired.

The number and variations of patient classification systems are unknown. Approximately 1,000 hospitals use some form of patient classification systems. The majority of these systems are based on a relatively limited number of approaches, similar to the criteria proposed by Conner, CASH, CSF Ltd., MEDICUS, and the University of Saskatchewan.[1] Developing a patient classification system that can be used to establish a staffing system certainly will not solve all of the staffing problems for a nursing administration. It can, however, provide a useful guide to establish an appropriate base line for staffing and for allocating personnel to meet daily needs as they fluctuate.[2]

A patient classification system is indeed a tool that, when appropriately implemented, can create more effective and productive utilization of nursing personnel resources. The effective utilization of nursing personnel does not guarantee the level of quality patient care but guarantees only a specified nurse-patient ratio. The measurement of patient care by patient outcome and a patient classification system, as well as by a coordinated staffing system, does not directly assure this quality of care, but rather it aids in providing adequate personnel to meet the basic needs of patients.

THREE BASIC STYLES OF PATIENT CLASSIFICATION SYSTEMS

There are three basic styles of patient classification systems. Nearly all systems are a combination of these basic formulas. These classification systems in turn are used to create a staffing system or pattern. The method or methods used for placing patients in a classification category define the style of system. The three basic systems of classification or acuity identification are (1) the descriptive, (2) the checklist, and (3) the time or relative value unit (RVU) standard.

The Descriptive Style

The descriptive acuity table is a concise, narrative approach in which the nurse places the patient into the category that best describes the level or intensity of care that the patient is receiving. With a descriptive acuity system, the patient does not have to qualify for all routines or procedures listed in one section in order to be placed in a specific category, but the category that most closely describes the care received is the category assigned to the patient. Exhibits 8-1, 8-2, and 8-3 show examples of a descriptive style of a patient acuity system.

Exhibit 8-1 Descriptive Style of Patient Classification—Subjective Classification

I. A. Self-care postop open heart patients—independent ambulation, self-care for bathing.
   B. Post-cardiac cath patients without complications—awaiting discharge that day.
   C. Self-care patients awaiting surgery for a future day.

II. A. Uncomplicated post open heart patients—require little or no assistance with ambulation. Partial bath. Daily weights. TED stockings.
   B. MI patients—bath assistance; little or no ambulation assistance; I & O; daily weights.
   C. Open heart patients the day of surgery—require preop care, support, teaching.
   D. Preop surgical patients who transfer to ICU after surgery including PTA's day of procedure.

III. A. Complicated post surgical patients—those requiring IV, tube care, wound care, frequent vital signs, assist for ambulation, positioning, assist with bathing.
   B. Cardiac cath patients on day of procedure—requiring preop and postop care the same day. Short-term bed rest.

IV. A. Patients requiring complete care—complete bathing, frequent skin care, feeding, bed rest requiring bedpan, urinal assistance, positioning assistance.

Source: Reprinted with permission of Nursing Department, St. Mary's Hospital, San Francisco, California.

The main problem with the descriptive style is the subjectivity of the nurse's interpretation of the patient's degree of illness. A patient classification system must be reliable; the system, when interpreted and completed by a number of individuals, must reflect the same results. If the category assigned to the patient is interpreted differently by individual nurses, as can easily happen with the descriptive style, the figures reported to the staffing office may result in a wide range of requested nurse-to-patient ratios. For example, if one nurse feels that 4 of the 20 patients on the unit belong in category IV of the descriptive style, while another nurse evaluates that 8 of the same 20 patients belong in category IV according to the same descriptive system, the nursing staffing office will assign additional personnel to the nurse who indicates 8 category IV patients. If nurse 2 is correct, it will be reflected in the nursing hours for that shift and consequently in the nursing hours per patient day meeting the budget requirements. But if nurse 2 has padded the system because of its subjective nature and ease for padding, then the nursing hours for the shift as well as for the 24-hour day would be high.

In order for any classification system to be reliable, all nursing personnel must classify the patient based on similar criteria and use the system in the same manner. Since this is usually difficult to accomplish with the descriptive style, many nursing administrations have moved from this subjective approach to patient assessments. Although the descriptive style is a quick-check guideline for assigning a patient to a category or level of care, the subjectivity of the approach and the inconsistency in categorizing patients seem to outweigh the advantage of a time-saving system of patient classification.

Exhibit 8-2 Descriptive Style of Patient Classification System

LEVEL OF CARE AREA OF CARE	CATEGORY I MINIMAL	CATEGORY II MODERATE	CATEGORY III EXTENSIVE	CATEGORY IV INTENSIVE
A. ACTIVITY	Up ad lib Bathes self Feeds self Cares for own personal hygiene	Up with assistance Assist with bath, meals, personal hygiene	Complete bed rest Complete bed rest with personal hygiene Needs to be fed, tube feed	Completely dependent Unconscious
B. TREATMENTS	Routine vital signs Preparation for test and/or procedures	Vital signs q4h or less Clinitest—AC & HS I & O Dressgs change 1 × /shift Catheter care Non-sterile hot packs Sitz baths	Vital and/or neuro signs q4h Seizure precautions Dressgs 2 × /shift or more Sterile procedures Isolation TCH q4h or more Suctioning/maintain a patent airway Continuous IV Special procedure, i.e., CVP Major surgery 24 hr post op	Vital and/or neuro signs q2h or more often Reverse isolation Dressgs changes q2h or more Active hemorrhaging Active seizuring within past 24 hours Category III criteria in addition to being confused or combative
C. MEDICATIONS	All medications qid or less often and PRN or STAT	All medications qid or more often excluding IVs	IV medications Hyperalimentation Control of refractory diabetes	IV additives, which require close monitoring
D. EQUIPMENT	No equipment other than PRN	Not more than 2 of the following tubes with routine care: Foley, T-Tube, Hemovac, Naso-gastric Cardiac monitoring— no arrhythmias in last 24 hours	Two or more tubes from Category II & ureteral CVP Dialysis shunt Continuous bladder irrig. Murphy drips Tracheotomy & laryngectomy Ostomies, chest tubes Cardiac monitoring	Ventilator-monitors Tracheotomy or laryngectomy, first 24h postop Vascular and/or chest cases, first 24h postop Peritoneal dialysis
E. TEACHING AND EMOTIONAL SUPPORT	Brief explanations Understands readily Communicates readily	Reinforcement of initial teaching	Teaching of resistive pts. Care & support of patients with severe emotional reactions Unable to communicate needs Initial teaching of patient and significant other	More extensive Category III teaching Death and dying aspect for patient and/or significant others

Source: Reprinted with permission of Nursing Department, Jo Ellen Smith Memorial Hospital, F. Edward Hebert Hospital, New Orleans.

Exhibit 8-3 Descriptive Style of Patient Classification

Category I

Minimal nursing care is provided primarily by assistants to the registered nurse under her general supervision.

1. Ambulatory
2. Feeds self
3. Bathes self
4. Minimal treatments, preps, etc.
5. Minimal medications
6. No deviation from acceptable behavior patterns

Category II

Moderate nursing care is provided primarily by assistants to the registered nurse and under her general supervision.

1. Ambulates with help
2. Assist with feeding
3. Assist with bathing
4. Moderate amount of treatment, preps, and/or supervision of self-treatment
5. Moderate amount of medications, routine IV therapy
6. Routine postoperative care
7. Isolation
8. Some deviation from acceptable behavior patterns

Category III

Acute nursing care is provided partially by registered nurse and always under her close supervision.

1. Complete bed rest
2. Constant observation
3. Requires life-sustaining measures
4. Frequent treatments, vital signs, suctioning, etc.
5. Frequent medications, intensive IV therapy, hyperalimentation, CVP lines, etc.
6. Unconsciousness
7. Totally dependent on nursing personnel for service
8. Postoperative and postanesthesia complications
9. Severe deviation from acceptable behavior patterns

Source: Reprinted with permission of Nursing Department, Ojai Valley Community Hospital, Ojai, California.

The Checklist Style

The checklist style of an acuity table divides the descriptions of care routines into activity groups such as eating, grooming, excretion, etc. By use of the checklist style, a judgment must be made for each patient in each activity grouping. The acuity levels of all the activities are then tallied; the total number of points assigned to the patient should reflect the category in which the patient will be placed. This method of patient classification is used to identify the patients either daily or by shift.

Exhibit 8-4 is an example of a checklist mode of acuity table. Although somewhat more specific, the checklist method, like the descriptive method, lends itself to subjective interpretation by those assigning the acuity points.

Exhibit 8-4 illustrates a patient classification system based on the checklist method; it was implemented in the med-surg unit of a 99-bed acute-care hospital. In this method each patient is assigned an acuity value in one of the eight categories of patient care: meals, grooming, excretion, activity, behavior, teaching, treatments, and medications. These values are not determined by any time-and-motion studies; rather, a random unit value is assigned to a task according to only an estimated length of time needed to complete the procedure or task; i.e., activities in category II take more time than activities in category I, and activities in category III take more nursing time than those in category II. The total time value then places the patient into a specific level of acuity, with level IV patients requiring the most time-consuming care.

At the hospital where this system was implemented, it was determined that nurses on different shifts could carry different patient loads. For example, on the day shift one nurse could be responsible for 60 to 70 units; on the evening shift one nurse could be responsible for 78 to 84 units; and on the night shift one nurse could be responsible for 85 to 99 units. It was determined that the number of units for which a nurse could reasonably assume responsibility was based on staffing that provides for a unit secretary and a nursing assistant (nurse aide). On the day and evening shifts, if a nursing assistant is unavailable, it becomes necessary to decrease each nurse's unit load by 8 to 10. If a unit secretary is unavailable, it is necessary to decrease the nurse's unit load by 5 units.

On the night shift the unit secretary and unit assistant positions are incorporated. Therefore, if this individual's role of a combined unit secretary and nursing assistant position were not available, the nurse's unit load would need to be decreased by 10 to 15 units per nurse. It was also determined that as the percentage of high acuity patients increased (15 percent or more), staffing needs would also be adjusted upward. For example, if a unit has 30 patients with a total acuity of 300 units or an average patient acuity of 10, many of those patients would be able to do much of their basic self-care. If, however, a unit has 15 patients with a total acuity of 300 units, the average patient acuity would be 20. This would imply, without

Exhibit 8-4 Checklist Style of Patient Classification

UNIT: ______________________

SHIFT: ______________________

DATE: ______________________

EVALUATION: ______________________

Instructions:

Check ( ) applicable statement for each classification in the appropriate patient column. Add total points to place patient in a category.

Total Points	*Category*
0 - 11	I
12 - 21	II
22+ - 30	III
30+ -	IV

		ROOM								
		AGE								
		PATIENT								
		Acuity Level								
EATING	Self-Care	1								
	Help Setting Up	2								
	Feed—Tube Feed	3								
	Feed with Problem Freq. Tube Feedings	4								
GROOM	Self-Bed Bath	1								
	Complete Care	2								
	Complete Care Problems	3								
EXCRET	Self-Care	1								
	Needs Help	2								
	Needs Frequent Help	3								
	Incontinent	4								
ACTIVITY	Ambulatory	1								
	Amb. with Help	2								
	Amb. or Turn with 2	3								
	Freq. Amb. with Help Complicating Apparatus	4								
BEHAVIOR	Alert—Oriented	1								
	Mildly Confused	2								
	Restraints—Confused	3								
	Demanding/Psychotic	4								

Exhibit 8-4 continued

		ROOM								
		AGE								
		PATIENT								
		Acuity Level								
TEACHING	Routine	1								
	Reinforcement	2								
	New Detailed Emotional Support	3								
	Communication Barrier	4								
TREATMENT	Routine Bedside Equipment	1								
	Cath Care Sitz—Moist. Comp.	2								
	Traction Decubitus Care	3								
	Freq. Suction—Tubes Wound Irrig. (Several)	4								
MEDICATION	Routine	1								
	Topical Ointments; Pre-Post OP/KVO IVs	2								
	8 IV/IVPB Many Meds PO	3								
	Freq. PRNs & IVPB Combination of Meds	4								
	Transfusion/TPN									
	Total Patient Acuity:									

looking at the specific acuity of each patient, that the majority of patients could not do much care for themselves in any category. This situation calls for more personalized, complex nursing care, which requires more of the nurse's time.

There are a number of problems with this method of patient classification system. First and foremost, no time-and-motion studies were done with this method to determine the actual time values before assigning a determining figure or relative value unit to the task. Rather, activities were randomly categorized into levels of care, i.e., level I, level II, level III, and level IV. This system leaves room for subjectivity on the part of the nurse assigning the acuity level to the individual patient. Another problem was that as the nurse's total patient unit load decreased, more nursing staff would be required to provide care for the increased patient units. Many nursing administrations are constantly dealing with the nursing shortage; they obtain additional nursing help through either registry or outside contract services. This continues to be an even more complex problem than that of merely determining the patient's acuity level.

Time or Relative Value Unit Style

The time standard or relative value unit (RVU) system employs a number of activities and aspects of patient care, which receive a value unit, usually a unit measure of time. Activities are then totaled so that the patient can be placed into a category, such as category I, category II, category III, or category IV. Some systems of relative value unit methods total the activities exclusively according to the direct care ordered by the physician on the patient chart rather than combining the nursing and medical team care, which may be charted in the patient's medical record.

Relative value unit systems vary greatly in complexity. Verification, review, and revision based on accumulated statistics, daily reports, and staff nurses' input must occur so that the most appropriate system is developed for the unique needs of each facility.

Exhibit 8-5 is an example of a time or relative value unit method for patient classification systems. Exhibit 8-5 is the classification system detailed throughout the book.

BENEFITS OF A PATIENT CLASSIFICATION SYSTEM

The hospital's nursing staff as well as patients themselves benefit from a patient classification system. Some of the benefits unique to each group are more obvious than others. From a patient's point of view, the purpose of a patient classification system is to categorize patients objectively according to the most selective method available, taking into account the individual needs of the patient. The patient,

Exhibit 8-5 Time or Relative Value Unit Method for Patient Classification System

	DATE		ACUITY ASSESSMENT
BATH		1	Sitz Bath
		1	Self Care / Shower / Tub
		2	Partial Bath
		3	Complete Bed Bath
		5	Complete Bed Bath w/Diff. Pt.
		1	Shampoo
DIET		1	NPO / Feeds Self
		2	Assist. w/Tray
		3	Feed Patient
		4	Difficult Feeder or Tube Feeding
		5	Keofeed
		7	Difficult Feeder and Tube Feeding
MOBILITY		0	Amublatory / B.R.P.
		1	Dangle
		2	Active / Passive R.O.M.
		2	B.P.R. w/Help X per Shift
		2	Chair w/Help X per Shift
		2	Commode w/Help X per Shift
		3	Ambulate w/Help
		3	Bedrest/Turn & Position O 2H
MONITOR		1	Cast & C.S.M.T. Check/Pulse Check
		1	Weight · Bathscale ☐ or Bedscale ☐
			Neuro Check Q ____
			T.P.R. · B.P. Q ____
			(Give one pt. for each V.S. or N.S. Check/Shift)
		1	Telemetry / Monitor
NEUR		0	Comatose
		1	Restrain
		2	Confused – Noncombative
		5	Confused – Combative
VENT.		1	Chest Tube (DC'D /)
		1	Oxygen
		1	Cough and Deep Breath
		2	Oral Suctioning
		2	Chest Tube / Emerson Pump
		3	Nasopharyngeal Suctioning
		4	Trach Suctioning and Care
		5	Respirator
OTHER		0	K Pad
		1	Foot Cradle
		1	Overhead Frame
		0	Sheepskin
		1	Egg Crate Mattress
		1	TEDS
		2	Hypothermia Blanket
		1	Ice Collar
		1	Voice Rest

	DATE		ACUTIY ASSESSMENT
G.I.		1	N. G. Suction
		1	N. G. Irrigation (Routine)
		1	Stool Specimen
		2	Colostomy / Ileal Care
		3	Enemas Till Clear
		6	N. G. Lavage (Active Bleed)
URINARY		0	Foley Catheter: Cath (DC'D /). Check time and amount of each voiding until (/).
		1	Strain Urine
		2	S. & A. Q ____
		1	Hemastix
		1	Quantitive Urine Collection
		1	Foley Care
		1	T.U.R. Foley Irrigation
		1	Clamp Foley
		2	Catheter to be Changed (/)
		2	Straight Catheterization
		2	I. & O.
		3	I. and O. 2H or Greater
			Incont. ( ) times/shift. Give 2 per incont.
		3	Cont. Bladder Irrigation
DRESSING		1	Simple Dressing Change
		1	Sterile Compress
		1	Reinforce Dressing or Check Q H
		2	Simple Decubitus Care
		3	Complex Dressing Change
		4	Subclavian / Swan Ganz Drsng Change
		5	Complex Decubitus Care
TEACH		3	Teaching Home Care, Discharge Planning (10 - 25 min. / Shift)
		7	Emotional Needs / Family Problems (1/2 - 1 hr. / Shift)
		9	Intensive Teaching (– 1 hr. / Shift)
DRAIN		0	Clips / Sutures (DC'D /)
		0	Penrose Drian (DC'D /)
		1	Hemovac (DC'D /)
		1	Jackson Pratt (DC'D /)
		1	X-Ray Procedure
		1	Nuclear Med. Procedure
		1	Cardiology Procedure
TRA.		3	Traction
P.T.		0	Physical Therapy

	DATE		ACUITY ASSESSMENT
ISOLA		3	Respiratory
		3	Enteric
		4	Wound & Skin
		7	Strict / Reverse
LINES		2	Arterial Line
		2	T. P. N.
		2	A. V. Shunt
		4	Swan Ganz
		4	Cardiac Output
		5	I. C. P.
I.V. MEDS.		3	Lidocaine
		3	Heparin
		3	Aminophylline
		3	Blood Products
		3	Chemo Therapy
		2	IVAC c̄ KCL
I.V. MEDS		5	Dopamine
		5	Nipride
		5	Isuprel
		5	Aramine
SITE		0	H. P. Inserted
		2	H. P. Change Due
		0	I. V. Inserted
		2	I. V. Change Due
MEDS		1	1 - 3 / Shift (Includes PRN)
		2	4 - 6 / Shift
		3	7 - 9 / Shift
		4	10 or more / Shift
IVS		2	Cont. I. V. Observation
		1	Change 1 Bottle / Shift
			__Piggyback/Shift. One pt. per Piggyback/Shift
		2	1 - 3 I.V. Push Meds / Shift
		3	4 - 6 I.V. Push Meds / Shift
R.T.		0	Respiratory Therapy

DATE	ACUITY
SIGNATURE	

then, benefits from such a classification system in that the nursing care delivered is more consistent because some predictions can be made about the care required.

From a nurse's point of view, the purpose of the patient classification system is to allow a nursing administration some meaningful way of staffing a nursing unit based on an objective approach to classifying a patient. With a patient classification system, staffing a nursing unit can be accomplished with a more certain degree of accuracy. It is the responsibility of the nursing administration to provide an objective patient classification system that can be the guideline for sound nurse staffing. Encouraging staff nurses to assist with the creation, implementation, and revision of the patient classification system helps staff nurses to recognize themselves as an integrated part of the nursing department. This approach also improves morale among the nursing staff.

Although variations of patient classification systems are numerous, they seem to be based generally on three common styles. A patient classification system must be designed and adapted to meet the specific needs of the hospital in which it is going to be implemented. When choosing the style or method of patient classification system for a particular hospital, the nursing administration must make the classification system meaningful to the nursing staff who will be delivering the care, while at the same time realistic in achieving nursing care goal hours. A customized classification system based on objective guidelines enables the nursing administration to utilize most effectively and efficiently the key resources within the nursing department—the nursing care staff—to their ultimate capacity.

While no patient classification system is without problems, a number of systems are functioning effectively in hospitals. No matter how well a system is working, there is always the need to review, revise, and justify that system.

NOTES

1. Phyllis Giovannetti, "Understanding Patient Classification Systems," *Journal of Nursing Administration,* February 1979, p. 4.
2. Ibid.

Chapter 9

Factors Affecting Patient Classification Systems

OBJECTIVES

Following completion of this chapter the reader will be able to:

- identify the factors that affect and impact a patient classification system and
- give examples of how these factors may affect the patient classification system.

Before a patient classification system can be developed for a particular facility, the nursing administration must be cognizant of the factors that influence such systems. Besides the federal and state regulations (such as Medicare, Joint Commission on Accreditation of Hospitals) that affect classification systems, several other factors must be considered. Institutional factors, the medical department, the nursing department, and the patient population also define to a degree some parameters of a patient classification system.

INSTITUTIONAL FACTORS

Type of Hospital

Is the facility teaching or nonteaching? If it is a teaching hospital with medical students, then the nursing staff may not be required to spend as much time assisting with procedures. On the other hand a teaching hospital exclusively for nursing students may require the nursing staff to devote a substantial amount of time to education and student supervision.

Size of Hospital

Is the facility large or small? Larger hospitals tend to group patients according to diagnosis and medical specialty. Consequently the nursing staff develop their expertise in given areas; smaller hospitals cannot group patients in the same manner, which requires each nurse to be a jack of all trades. Furthermore, fluctuations in patient acuity and census appear to impact smaller facilities more noticeably than larger facilities.

Characteristics of Hospital Administration

Is the hospital administration a cohesive group? Is the nursing administration recognized and adequately represented as an integral part of this group? Does the hospital administration respect and understand the practice of the nursing process? Favorable replies to these questions provide the nursing department with a sense of autonomy and belonging within the hospital. This in turn has a positive effect on the nursing staff, for they will be able to conceptualize health care from more than a nursing perspective. The incentive to work diligently and to work within specific guidelines becomes validated with adequate support and recognition.

Budgetary Source and Constraints

Is the nursing administration preparing, developing, and maintaining the responsibility for its own budgetary process? What justifications are needed to support variances from budget? It is unrealistic to be held accountable for a process that was developed without nursing input. With this approach the nursing staff will say: "Why bother with acuities? The hospital administration doesn't care. It doesn't even let the nursing administration develop its own budget."

Technology

Does the medical staff practice sophisticated medicine? Highly technical equipment poses several constraints. The equipment needs space for use and storage; it needs to be operated and maintained by specially trained individuals; and it needs to be updated on an ongoing constant basis. Use of highly technical equipment usually mandates that nurses too be highly trained, as in the case of critical care nursing.

The Physical Plant

Does the facility enjoy the luxury of offering all private rooms or provide a combination of private, semiprivate, and ward accommodations? If it provides the latter, then valuable nursing time is frequently exhausted in assigning rooms—smoker versus nonsmoker, older versus younger, surgical versus medical, isolation, etc. Is the facility a high-rise building, where the staff are spread out and must therefore contend with periodic nonfunctioning elevators? Does the facility utilize a conveyor belt or pneumatic tube system that provides safe and efficient delivery of supplies and drugs or does the nursing staff function as the delivery system?

Specialty Services

Does the facility provide psychiatric, obstetric, and pediatric specialty services? These services require especially trained personnel and may require a separate patient classification system from medical/surgical units. How do respiratory therapy and physical therapy departments function? Do they merely provide patient service and instruction and then depend on nursing for follow-up? Do the cardiology department and the laboratory provide services 24 hours a day or does the nursing staff run electrocardiograms (EKGs) and draw arterial blood gases when these departments are closed?

THE MEDICAL DEPARTMENT

Characteristics of the Medical Staff

Do the medical staff exhibit a high level of enthusiasm? Are they eager to learn new techniques and willing to teach? Do they keep pace with medical knowledge and standards of practice within the community? How do the medical staff perceive nursing practice: as an equal component to the medical staff? as part of the team? What are their work patterns: rounds early in the morning or late in the evening? rounds once a day with an energetic group of medical students and nursing students? Is the nursing staff encouraged and welcomed to participate in rounds with the physicians?

Privileges in Other Facilities

Denial of medical practice privileges by one facility may directly affect another facility, its method of staffing, and patient acuity. For instance, a physician focusing on Medicare patients was recently denied privileges in a large metropolitan hospital. Consequently a neighboring facility absorbed most of these patients, who required more nursing time to deliver adequately the care mandated by the particular standards. Because this facility did not routinely admit such a large proportion of time-consuming patients with a multitude of problems, the nursing administration did not have a patient classification system and staffing pattern capable of addressing and adequately caring for these patients.

Levels of Expertise

Are the physicians clinically competent to manage the patient? If not, are the physicians willing to refer the patient to a specialist/consultant? In the absence of such a referral do the nursing staff assume the responsibility for managing the care of the cardiac patient because the physician is not a cardiologist? How does a patient needing, but not receiving, psychiatric assistance affect the nursing staff and the staffing patterns?

Therapeutic Modalities

Generally do the medical staff emphasize a liberal approach to health, namely, performing the latest procedures and using the newest medications, or is a more conservative approach emphasized? How much nursing time is utilized in assisting certain physicians with technical procedures and complex treatments?

Awareness of Nursing and Nursing Modalities

Are the medical staff educated to the various styles of nursing care delivery, i.e., team leading, total patient care, and primary nursing concepts? Are the medical staff threatened by nurses with advanced preparation or do they welcome nurses in expanded roles? Lack of awareness of nursing modalities and passive participation in a nurse's potential may adversely affect patient care. Are the medical staff aware of the value of discharge planning and supportive of follow-up in the home? Without awareness and support, hospitalization may be prolonged, thereby adding to the responsibility of the nursing staff; valuable time will be expended caring for a patient who could be discharged from the hospital if only the physician would write the order.

THE NURSING DEPARTMENT

Characteristics of the Nursing Staff

Is the nursing staff comprised of licensed staff exclusively or is it a combination of RNs, LVNs, aides, and orderlies? What biopsychosocial influences affect the staff? Are the staff young, inexperienced, and readily adaptable to change? Are they older, experienced, and possibly set in their ways? What is the educational background of the nursing staff? How experienced is the middle management team in regard to leadership? What social and ethnic backgrounds influence the staff? Are many of them graduates of foreign schools? What is the ratio of full-time, part-time, and on-call/per-diem staff employed? What is the average monthly registry utilization? Considering licensed versus unlicensed staff, what is the ratio between RN and LVN staff? All these vital factors must be considered when developing a patient classification system.

The Nursing Domain

What services are solely the responsibility of the nursing department: critical care, emergency department, medical/surgical units, outpatient services, volunteer services? Does the nursing department become extensible during certain hours of the day? In other words does nursing service make sandwiches when the dietary department is closed, prepare intravenous injections (IVs) when the pharmacy is closed, and empty wastebaskets when housekeeping is closed?

Flexibility

Is the nursing administration flexible and open to new ideas and changing concepts? Is the nursing administration content with the status quo and afraid to rock the boat or is it open-minded and challenged by change processes in a turbulent environment?

Management Style

Is nursing service a centralized or decentralized department? Is one individual the decision maker or are decisions the result of a group process? Is the nursing administration top-heavy? Is the middle management team supportive but independent?

Teaching Programs

Is the facility associated with a school of nursing? Does the facility offer a preceptorship program or is education the sole responsibility of the inservice department?

PATIENT POPULATION

Characteristics

What are the socioeconomic status, the ethnic background, and the age of the patients utilizing the services of the facility?

Expectations of Care

Does the patient population possess sophisticated knowledge of what should be provided in health care or does the patient population think that the doctors and nurses know best?

Diagnosis of General Level of Health

Does the patient population seek medical advice on a routine basis? Does the patient population recognize the need for preventative medical care as well as palliative and curative health care? Lack of preventative health care due to depressed economic conditions or poor accessibility to a facility may increase the number of medical problems encountered. In general a low level of health and the subsequent medical problems increase the need for medical and nursing assistance.

Geographical Location

Do the patient needs reflect the geographical location? Is the facility located in a resort area? Does the patient population peak during certain seasons? For instance, skiing accidents in the winter and allergy attacks in the spring may impact facilities in resort areas to a greater extent than facilities in large metropolitan cities. Furthermore, environmentally related problems such as smog, hurricane, or tornado must be taken into consideration when attempting to develop a strategic staffing plan.

Turnover

What are the turnover rates—above or below the national averages (24 percent)? What are the reasons for turnover? Is the staff attracted to the facility seasonally for limited periods of time for recreational or educational purposes? Is the facility able to absorb students from nearby schools of nursing? What is the local competition?

Nursing Resources

Are resources available to the staff for inservice education? Are continuing education credits offered on the premises?

Standards of Care

Who establishes standards of nursing care practice? How often are they reviewed and revised? Are they clearly written and available to all staff members?

How many standards are informal and unwritten? Are the standards of care realistic and measurable? Are they grounded in subservience, servitude, and nurturing?

Presence of Unionization and Professional Activity

Is the facility unionized? What do the contracts mandate? Does the nursing administration honor the contract explicitly? What is the emotional climate between nursing administration and the nursing staff after a contract has been negotiated and ratified?

These factors are not all-inclusive. However, they should provide some thought-provoking ideas and questions. The number and kinds of factors, as well as their relative importance, vary from facility to facility, from unit to unit, and from year to year. It cannot be overemphasized that every institution must address these factors, and many more, before and during the development of a patient classification system and subsequent staffing system. Once developed, both the patient classification system and the staffing system cannot remain static because the components of both systems—patients and nurses—are forever changing. In addition to developing and analyzing such systems, nursing administrators and staff nurses must be willing to review and revise these systems constantly. This ongoing process assures input, output, and feedback for all concerned in maintaining quality standards of nursing practice and patient care.

Chapter 10

Yesterday's Patient Classification System

OBJECTIVES

Following completion of this chapter the reader will be able to:

- identify factors affecting this patient classification system and
- describe the process of change in relationship to the conditions necessary for successful change to take place (discussed in Chapter 5).

A small hospital, nestled in the rolling hills of Northern California, was constructed in the mid-1960s and is privately owned. It is centrally located in a serene residential community. The patient population consists of local residents as does much of the hospital personnel. The physician staff consists primarily of family practitioners with a few specialists. Their services are generally divided among their own well-established practices and three centrally located medical facilities. The hospital is a teaching institution with educational services limited to RN students at a nearby community college. The nursing staff is comprised of an essential minimum of registered nurses dispensing medications and maintaining IVs, a zealous group of licensed vocational nurses functioning as aides and chomping at the bit to do more, and an overabundance of nurses' aides doing bedside, hands-on nursing.

In the late 1960s and early 1970s team nursing was in vogue as an appropriate nursing modality at this hospital, which catered to a rather healthy, middle-aged community. Acute critical care nursing and trauma medicine had not yet been introduced.

But in the mid-1970s things began to change in this location. Single-family dwellings, condominiums, and townhouses were taking root in underdeveloped areas of the community and adjacent areas. Eager to purchase affordable homes and settle, people flocked to this area. Shopping complexes, schools, and office buildings were erected to meet the needs of the growing community. As the population within the community increased, so did the patient population. Simultaneously there was an influx of young physicians educated in medical schools dedicated to practicing high-powered medicine. Like their predecessors, they too believed in preventative, curative, and palliative medicine. In order to practice such standards of medicine, they relied heavily on the newest diagnostic equipment and procedures. Before long, the small facility found itself sporting the latest fashion in CAT scanners and critical care equipment. The staff was a proud group—proud of the zealous and enthusiastic medical staff, the dedicated and hard-working nursing staff, and the high-tech facility.

JCAH REVIEW

In the late 1970s reality struck. In 1977 the Joint Commission on Accreditation of Hospitals was invited to visit the facility. JCAH challenged, and rightly, the patient classification and staffing systems. It questioned the lack of licensed professional personnel in relation to the status of the patients. The age-old problem of care plans surfaced. There was no concrete patient classification system, established staffing pattern, or measurable, realistic patient care plans that were completed with regularity. Patient kardexes hardly allowed enough space for urgent treatments and medicines let alone space for measurable, realistic care plans. In essence the classification system, staffing system, and care plans were rather vague and incongruent.

EXPLORING CLASSIFICATION SYSTEMS

Shortly after the departure of the JCAH team, the nursing administration developed a plan of action. Unit coordinators and inservice personnel would research and develop an updated, all-inclusive patient kardex while the nursing administrator would explore adaptable patient classification systems. After months of brainstorming and compromise, a suitable patient kardex was developed, printed, and implemented in the nursing units (Exhibit 10-1). A few months later this new patient kardex was expanded to include the patient classification system that most suited the facility. The instructional directive that accompanied this new patient classification system stressed the importance of identifying patient intensity or acuity precisely and the impact such intensity or acuity had on staffing systems.

In other words this patient classification system was designed to supply the nursing administration with a method to allocate adequate and appropriately skilled staff to meet the predetermined standards of nursing care. Basically this particular system mandated that each patient be categorized according to certain subjective criteria. To determine the actual acuity level of a patient, one simply

Exhibit 10-1 Nursing Care Plan and Patient Kardex

NURSING CARE PLAN

GOAL: FORM DH-505-07

ACTIVITY AND DATE	NURSING PROBLEM AND NEEDS	APPROACH
BED REST ______		
CHAIR ______		
B. R. P. ______		
WITH HELP ______		
AMBULATORY ______		
WITH HELP ______		
WEIGHT ______		
FEED ______		
RESTRAINTS ______		
SIDE RAILS ______		
BATH ______	NAME AND PHONE NUMBER OF PERSON TO NOTIFY	

ADM. DATE	ADM. DX.	MEDS PHARMACY ☐		DIET AND FLUIDS	ALLERGY
SURGERY DATE	SURGICAL PROCEDURE	AGE	RELIGION		

Exhibit 10-1 continued

				PENDING PROCEDURES	
BEGIN	P. R. N. MEDICATIONS	D. C.	DATE	LABORATORY	SLIP SENT
			DATE	X-RAY	SLIP SENT
	H. S. MEDICATIONS				

BEGIN	ROUTINE MEDICATIONS	HOURS DUE	D.C.	BEGIN	TREATMENTS	D.C.

ROOM	NAME (LAST FIRST MIDDLE) M W S D	HOSP. NO.	PHYSICIAN AND PHONE NUMBER

Source: Reprinted with permission of Doctors Hospital of Pinole, Pinole, California.

totaled the designated categories and divided by 4. The subjective criteria has two advantages. First, they allowed each patient to be assessed in a rapid manner; therefore valuable time was not wasted. Second, each nurse was allowed to assess patients according to personal biases, judgments, or interpretations. While the nursing staff was a rather compliant group who diligently assessed their patients every day, this system soon created havoc with the nursing administration, particularly as it attempted to interpret and justify the results and staff accordingly. The major disadvantage was that this system had no built-in mechanism to assure accuracy, realism, or accountability. Consequently allocation of staff was inappropriate and the quality of care was inadequate (Exhibits 10-2 and 10-3).

Role of Staff Allocation

Quality nursing care is directly dependent on appropriate allocation of staff. Without proper allocation several problems arise. The following gamut of complaints is frequently registered with the nursing administration. Nurses complain that they are overworked, underpaid, and understaffed. Patients complain that they are ignored or unattended. Physicians complain that they can't find a nurse, the chart, or the patient. Everyone wants and needs help.

As the complaints escalate in the absence of any resolution toward the staffing problem, additional, complicating developments evolve. Nurses seek the support and assistance of their organized associations, patients write derogatory letters to the hospital administration promising never to return (even for a visit), and physicians ally to form a nursing advisory committee infamously designed to tell nursing exactly how to solve their problems properly. While the nurses association demands that more nurses be hired, the hospital administration forwards the patient letters to the nursing administration, and the nursing advisory committee merely recommends that adding more staff will solve the problem. The end result is that these complaints filter through to the executive committee—and the ultimatum for change is demanded.

CASH System

The new staffing system was vetoed by nursing administration. Lacking a certain amount of confidence at this point, nursing administration enlisted the services of a professional management engineering firm to develop a method of measuring nursing workloads and relating them to specific needs. The Commission for Administrative Services in Hospitals (CASH) presented a patient classification system. The package created conflict within the nursing staff but allowed the nursing administration to improve control over staff allocation. The nursing staff found the CASH system tedious and time-consuming. In their judgment CASH was useless because they saw no appreciable increase in the number of staff as patient acuity rose.

Exhibit 10-2 Patient Care Plan

DOCTORS HOSPITAL - PINOLE

PATIENT CARE PLAN

CODE STATUS

ISOLATION:

ALLERGIES:

BRIEF MEDICAL HISTORY:

DISCHARGE PLANS:

DATE	NURSING DX/PROBLEM	GOAL (LONG & SHORT TERM)	NURSING ACTION

ADM. DATE		TO ICU/CCU	TO FLOOR	RELIGION	HOSP. NO.

ADM. DX:

CURRENT DX:

SURG. DATE	SURGICAL PROCEDURE	DATE	SPECIAL PROCEDURES

DIET:

Assist c̄ Tray

Feed

Tube Feedings

Fluids:

Exhibit 10-2 continued

	DATE	
BATH		Shower/Tub
		Partial
		Complete
		Sitz Bath
OBSERVATIONS		Weight Bedscale Bathscale
		TPR
		BP
		Neuro Checks
		Pedal Pulse Check
		Cast and CMST Check
		I & O Last BM
		Dressing Check
		Compresses
		K Pad
MOBILITY		Bedrest Dangle
		Chair
		BRP Help ☐
		Ambulate Help ☐
		Turn & Position
		Active/Passive ROM
		Leg Exercises
		Physical Therapy:

	DATE	
VENT		Cough & Deep Breath
		Cont. Mech. Aide Vent.
		Oral & Nasal Suctioning
		Oxygen
		Resp. Therapy
TREATMENTS		Clinitest and Acetest
		Colostomy Irrigation and Care
		Decubitus Care
		Eggshell Mattress
		Foot Cradle
		Overhead Frame & Trapeze
		Restraints
		Sheepskin
		Teds
		Telemetry/Monitor
		Trach Care
		Traction

	DATE	
TUBES		Foley Catheter
		Cath. Care
		Irrigate Foley
		Clamp Foley
		Cath. Change ☐
		Cath. Dc'd ☐ → Check
		Time & Amount of Each Voiding
		Chest Tube
		Chest Tube Milking
		Chest Tube Dc'd ☐
		Hemovac
		Jackson Pratt
		NG Tube
		Irrigate Ng Tube
		Ng Tube Dc'd ☐
		Penrose Drain Dc'd ☐
		Shunt
		Sutures Dc'd ☐
LINES		H. P. Insert ☐
		H. P. Change Due ☐
		IV Insert ☐
		IV Change Due ☐
		Other Lines:

BEGIN	ROUTINE MEDS	TIME	DC	BEGIN	PRN MEDICATIONS	TIME	DC
					H S MEDS		
				DATE	LAB		
				DATE	X-RAY		
				DATE	NUCLEAR MEDICINE		

RELATIVE & PHONE NUMBER		CONSULTING PHYSICIAN	
ROOM	NAME M.S. D.W.	AGE	PRIMARY PHYSICIAN	FORM DH 505-07

Source: Reprinted with permission of Doctors Hospital of Pinole, Pinole, California.

Exhibit 10-3 Acuity Assessment

DOCTORS HOSPITAL - PINOLE

PATIENT CARE PLAN

CODE STATUS

ISOLATION:

ALLERGIES:

BRIEF MEDICAL HISTORY:

DISCHARGE PLANS:

DATE	DX / PROBLEM	GOAL (LONG & SHORT TERM)	ACTION

ADM. DATE		TO ICU/CCU	TO FLOOR	RELIGION	HOSP. NO.

ADM. DX:

CURRENT DX:

SURG. DATE	SURGICAL PROCEDURE	DATE	SPECIAL PROCEDURES

DIET:

Assist c̄ Tray

Feed

Tube Feedings

Fluids:

	DATE	
B		Shower/Tub
A		Partial
T		Complete
H		Sitz Bath
O		Weight Bedscale Bathscale
B		TPR
S		BP
E		Neuro Checks
R		Pedal Pulse Check
V		Cast and CMST Check
A		I & O Last BM
T		Dressing Check
I		
O		Compresses
N		
S		
		K Pad
M		Bedrest Dangle
O		Chair
B		BRP Help ☐
I		Ambulate Help ☐
L		Turn & Position
I		Active/Passive ROM
T		Leg Exercises
Y		Physical Therapy:

	DATE	
V		Cough & Deep Breath
E		Cont. Mech. Aide Vent.
N		Oral & Nasal Suctioning
T		Oxygen
		Resp. Therapy
T		Clinitest and Acetest
R		Colostomy Irrigation and Care
E		Decubitus Care
A		Eggshell Mattress
T		Foot Cradle
M		Overhead Frame & Trapeze
E		Restraints
N		Sheepskin
T		Teds
S		Telemetry/Monitor
		Trach Care
		Traction

ACUITY ASSESSMENT

	1	2	3	4
Physical				
Medication/Treatments				
Observation				
Psycho/Social				
Instructional				

Date:__________
Nurse:__________

	DATE	
T		Foley Catheter
U		Cath. Care
B		Irrigate Foley
E		Clamp Foley
S		Cath. Change ☐
		Cath. Dc'd ☐ → Check
		Time & Amount of Each Voiding
		Chest Tube
		Chest Tube Milking
		Chest Tube Dc'd ☐
		Hemovac
		Jackson Pratt
		NG Tube
		Irrigate Ng Tube
		Ng Tube Dc'd ☐
		Penrose Drain Dc'd ☐
		Shunt
		Sutures Dc'd ☐
L		H. P. Insert ☐
I		H. P. Change Due ☐
N		IV Insert ☐
E		IV Change Due ☐
S		Other Lines:

Exhibit 10-3 continued

BEGIN	ROUTINE MEDS	TIME	DC

BEGIN	PRN MEDICATIONS	TIME	DC
	H S MEDS		

DATE	LAB

DATE	X-RAY

DATE	NUCLEAR MEDICINE

RELATIVE & PHONE NUMBER

CONSULTING PHYSICIAN

ROOM | NAME M.S. D.W. | AGE | PRIMARY PHYSICIAN

FORM DH 505-07

AREA OF CARE	CATEGORY I	CATEGORY II	CATEGORY III	CATEGORY IV
PHYSICAL	Feeds self or needs minimal assistance. Bathes & dresses self w/little help. Ambulates w/minimal or no assistance. Up to bathroom alone or w/ minimal assistance.	Needs some help and/or encouragement. May need meats cut & foods arranged. Needs some help w/bathing. BRP w/assistance.	Must be fed but is able to chew & swallow. Tube feedings. Participates minimally in bathing & grooming. Uses bedpan and/or urinal w/help. Occasionally incontinent (less than twice per shift). Turning & repositioning can usually be accomplished by one person.	Cannot feed self & has difficulty chewing & swallowing. Tube feedings q2h or more often. Totally dependent for cleanliness, grooming, excretory functions and position changes.
MEDS TREATMENTS	Routine meds not requiring pre or post evaluation. 2/shift or less. PRN meds not more than once/shift. Simple tests, procedure and/or treatments requiring 10 minutes or less in preparation and/or administration.	3-5 routine meds/shift. 2 or more PRN meds/shift. IV w/ or without meds. Routine monitoring. Bottle change not more than once/shift. Tests, procedures, and/or treatments requiring 10-30 minutes in preparation and/or administration. VS q4h or less often.	6-8 routine meds/shift. 2 or more PRN meds/shift. Complicated IVs. Bottle change more than once/shift; push med × 2/shift; IV controller in use. Tests, procedures and/or treatments requiring 30-60 minutes/shift. VS q 2-4 hours.	9 or more routine meds/shift. Life-sustaining meds requiring continuous monitoring & regulating. Complicated IVs. IVs to be started. Transfusions × 2 or more/shift. Tests, procedures and/or treatments requiring 60 minutes or more/shift. VS, outputs, etc., q2h or more/shift.
OBSERVATIONS	Routine VS. Mild symptoms of disease. In for diagnostic procedure, simple treatment and/or simple surgical procedures, traction, etc.	Moderate symptoms of disease. May have more than one illness. Extreme symptoms have subsided but symptoms still exist. Obviously ill but following usual course.	Acute symptoms of disease. May have more than one illness. Examples: Immediate post-head trauma, immediate post major surgery w/ drainage tubes, etc.	Seriously or critically ill; requires frequent observations. May or may not be terminal. Emergency therapeutic measures may be impending or under way.

Exhibit 10-3 continued

AREA OF CARE	*CATEGORY I*	*CATEGORY II*	*CATEGORY III*	*CATEGORY IV*
PSYCHO SOCIAL	No unusual or adverse emotional reactions. Appears adjusted to situation (family & patient). Special trips to provide emotional support requiring less than 10 minutes/shift.	Mild adverse reactions to illness. Needs support for depression. May be overly demanding. Special trips to provide emotional support requiring 10-20 minutes/shift.	Moderate adverse reactions to illness. Requires frequent observation & care for being demanding; confused; anxious; irritable; frightened; hostile; etc. (family and/or patient). Special trips to provide emotional support and/or to deal w/aforementioned requiring 20-60 minutes/shift.	Severe adverse reactions to illness. Unpredictable behavior requires close observation. May have severe symptoms of depression, disorientation, diliriums, hallucinations, hostility, etc. Special trips to provide emotional support and/or to deal w/the aforementioned requiring 60 minutes or more/shift.
			MAY BE PLACED IN THESE CATEGORIES ONLY IF CHARTED	
INSTRUCTIONAL	No specific teaching needs or teaching that can be conducted during the normal course of activities, i.e., during bed making time, while meds are being administered, etc.	Teaching requiring less than 10 minutes/shift (family and patient).	Teaching requiring 10-30 minutes/shift.	Teaching requiring more than 30 minutes/shift.
		MAY BE PLACED IN THESE CATEGORIES ONLY IF TEACHING IS RECORDED IN CHART AND ONLY IF TEACHING IS DONE BY ASSIGNED PERSONNEL		

Source: Reprinted with permission of Doctors Hospital of Pinole, Pinole, California.

Although CASH failed to provide a measurable justification system for increasing or decreasing staff numbers as patient or unit acuities increased and decreased, it was through CASH that the nursing administration began to look critically at the concept of staffing systems and patient acuity systems. In terms of sheer numbers of employees, theoretically the staff was adequate. However, there was a lack of licensed personnel necessary to deliver the quality of care mandated in conjunction with the quality of care that the physicians practiced and the quality of care that the patient warranted. Identifying and recognizing this fact would create position control, the backbone of all staffing systems.

In 1979 the JCAH review was repeated. While review was far from perfect, some improvement was shown in the area of patient classification and staffing systems. Immediately after the review, the nursing staff overtly rejected CASH and, as a result, subtly overlooked the daily assessment of each patient. The nursing administration was forced back to step 1. Complaints from patients, nurses, and physicians began to increase substantially. Suddenly, the nursing administration changed hands—and with it the direction of leadership.

SHARED CONCERNS

The life style changed drastically from this point. The new nursing administrator, assistant directors of nursing, and unit coordinators (formerly head nurses) were cordially invited to attend the nursing advisory committee meeting, a medical staff committee dedicated to solving nursing problems and thus improving patient care. The shared concerns were well-founded. Medications were not always administered on time, staffing was not always adequate, and changes in a patient's status were not always reported promptly to the physicians. In the eyes of some members of the medical staff these problems could be alleviated if more staff, but not necessarily licensed staff, were hired.

When concepts of total patient care and primary care were introduced and defined, the members of the nursing advisory committee strongly resisted. As one physician stated: "Nurses shouldn't be giving bed baths, they should be supervising. Hire more aides."

Perspectives misaligned, the nursing advisory committee didn't sympathize with the fact that the RN's span of control (18 patients and 2 to 3 staff members) was impossible to maintain if quality patient care were to be delivered. Actually the team nursing approach to patient care was merely a fragmented, inadequate approach; the RN rarely saw, let alone accurately assessed, patients. Because of the physicians' unfamiliarity with nursing modalities, it was difficult to convince the medical staff of the merits associated with total patient care and primary care. But it was of paramount importance for the nursing administration to maintain the decision-making power to choose the most feasible nursing modality for the institution. Finally it was agreed that a pilot program would be instituted, tested, and evaluated before a hospitalwide program was developed.

TOTAL PATIENT CARE

To introduce total patient care, two different plans had to be developed. Because the medical staff only half-heartedly supported the concept and because contractual agreements with professional associations influenced the process of organizational change, the nursing administration elected to introduce plan A, knowing that eventually plan B would have to be introduced if total patient care were to become a reality. Plan A was an evolutionary approach to change. Any particular unit and its regularly assigned staff would be selected to pilot this program. If this failed, as expected, plan B would be introduced, whereby personnel consciously committed to total patient care would be selected for the program.

The reader may be wondering why the nursing administration purposely implemented a plan of action doomed for failure: Contract agreements had mandated staff assignment and placement according to seniority and experience.

Consequently the apple cart could not be upset until a particular group of individuals had been given the opportunity to implement total patient care—and fail. Plan A failed because the concept of total patient care upset the status quo. Representing the status quo were those staff members dedicated to the concept of team nursing but, in order to survive and maintain employment in that particular unit, verbally supporting total patient care. However, total patient care required that RNs return to bedside, hands-on nursing while LVNs become inserviced and reeducated in skills, including drug administration. Hence, the roles of the nursing staff were to change. Although the status quo members verbally supported the concept, few were prepared to face this kind of change. The LVN staff wanted more money since they were expected to be doing more, while the RN staff fearfully wondered what RNs would be doing if not dispensing medications.

The details of plan B are unimportant at this point. Plan B succeeded because those individuals truly committed to the concept of total patient care, as opposed to mere survival, volunteered their services. Registered nurses seeking more intense patient contact and LVNs seeking to develop their potential and practice drug administration sought a working environment in which their desires could become a reality. Plan B provided any enthusiastic, concerned, and motivated individual the opportunity to practice total patient care. The group selected to implement plan B would be the same group of individuals who would unknowingly provide the nursing administration with the initial information necessary to develop an effective patient classification system.

Chapter 11

Methodology of the Current Patient Classification System

OBJECTIVES

Following completion of this chapter the reader will be able to:

- define patient care according to skill level and
- distribute patient assignments according to relative value units as opposed to the number of patients.

Initially, total patient care resolved several issues. Complaints from patients and physicians decreased, nursing errors and oversights became less frequent, and staff morale improved. Realistic, measurable, and personalized care plans began to be developed by the nursing staff. Even the daily patient assignment sheet (Exhibit 11-1) was replaced by a form that indicated the patient's name as well as the room number (Exhibit 11-2).

The nursing staff wanted the care that they delivered to be personalized and individualized. Hence, they viewed a patient classification system as a means of accomplishing this goal. They weren't content simply to know the similarities among their patients. They wanted to know the specific differences between patients—or the uniqueness of each patient—so that personalized and individualized care would be a reality and routine care could be avoided. They wanted the patient classification system to incorporate these differences, and they also wanted the differences reflected in the daily patient assignments. The nursing administration too wanted a patient classification system descriptive of the different, individual needs of the patient and reflective of the variable skill levels of the total staff of RNs, LVNs, and NAs.

Who would develop such a system: the nursing administration? the nursing staff? middle management? In the eyes of the staff, the nursing administration had

Exhibit 11-1 Daily Patient Assignment Sheet—Model A

WARD	DAILY ASSIGNMENT				DATE		
Team Leader	K. Smith RN				L. Jones RN		
Time	A. Silver LVN	B. Gold LVN	G. White NA	M. Black LVN	D. Green NA	H. Brown LVN	
	101 A 101 B 103 A 104 B 105 A 105 B	102 A 102 B 102 C 102 D 106 A 107 B	108 A 108 B 109 A 109 B 112 A 112 B	110 A 110 B 111 A 111 B 111 C 111 D	114 A 114 B 115 A 116 B 117 A 117 B	118 A 118 B 118 C 118 D 119 B 120 B	
Lunch							
Relief							
Group							

Team Conference

Source: Reprinted with permission of Nursing Department, Doctors Hospital of Pinole, Pinole, California.

Exhibit 11-2 Daily Patient Assignment Sheet—Model B

DATE: August 26, 1983 HEAD/CHARGE NURSE: JANET HENRY

NURSE	ACUITY	NURSE KATHY MILLER RN	ACUITY	NURSE JOAN RIDER LVN	ACUITY	NURSE MARGIE LESS RN	ACUITY	NURSE	ACUITY	NURSE	ACUITY
		633 Smith	22	637 Black	16	643 Little	10				
		638 Jones	10	642 White	8	644 Brown	6				
		IVs	2			IVs	2				
BREAKS & MEAL:		BREAKS & MEAL:		BREAKS & MEAL:		BREAKS & MEAL:		BREAKS & MEAL:		BREAKS & MEAL:	
TOTAL ACUITY		TOTAL ACUITY		TOTAL ACUITY		TOTAL ACUITY		TOTAL ACUITY		TOTAL ACUITY	

Source: Reprinted with permission of Nursing Department, Doctors Hospital of Pinole, Pinole, California.

already failed twice in its attempts to implement a patient classification system. Furthermore, since the nursing administration was often removed from bedside nursing, the general consensus was that it was incapable of accurately assessing the needs of the patients and the strengths and weaknesses of the staff. Why shouldn't help come from individuals most knowledgeable about the subject matter, namely, the unit coordinators and staff nurses? In other words, the base of participation should be broadened. A collaborative effort assures not only higher quality solutions to problems but also that behaviors and attitudes, once changed, remain changed. Through a teamsmanship attitude, people support what they help create.

DETERMINING PATIENT CARE

Unit coordinators and charge nurses agreed to meet weekly to discuss and develop the patient classification system that best suited their needs. During the first meeting the group was emphatic that two issues be agreed on. First, they wanted an objective system that left no room for subjective viewpoints and individual interpretations on the part of the nursing staff. Second, they wanted a system reflective of the patient clientele, the practicing medical staff, and the specific nursing staff. Before anything further could be developed, the group needed to determine exactly what was being done for patients and the time utilized to deliver set standards of care. Hence, nursing resorted to the time-and-motion study. The staff nurses who desired to participate in the total patient care project were also requested to participate in the time-and-motion study. The study was conducted over a two-week time span that incorporated activities from all three shifts. Exhibits 11-3 and 11-4 illustrate the manner in which these activities were recorded in detail.

After the time-and-motion study, the unit coordinators and charge nurses reviewed the data collected and grouped the activities according to categories (such as grooming, excretion, medications, etc.) and to relative value units. The relative value unit is a numerical value that represents a range of minutes needed to complete a particular task. (For example, 1 RVU = procedures and tasks requiring less than 6 minutes; 2 RVU = tasks taking 7 to 12 minutes; 3 RVUs = 13 to 18 minutes; 4 RVUs = 19 to 24 minutes; and 5 RVUs = procedures requiring more than 24 minutes.)

Grouping the activities according to categories was a fairly simple endeavor. On the other hand, defining RVUs was the most difficult part of the task. The initial approach was to determine the *exact* amount of time required to perform a specific task. For instance, did it take 10 minutes, 15 minutes, or 20 minutes to finish a complete bed bath? This approach came to an immediate halt when it became apparent that the exact amount of time required varied from one individual to the next. For example, although one nurse may be able to complete the task in 20 minutes, perhaps the same task can be expedited by a second in 15 minutes.

The second approach was then to determine an *average* amount of time required to perform any given task. For example, adding the total amount of time expended for complete bed baths from the time-and-motion study and then dividing by the number of examples yielded the *average* amount of time designated to that task. Once again, establishing an average amount of time was too limiting in that only one absolute figure would be defined. In essence, this approach was not much different than the initial approach.

The final and most successful approach determined a range of time realistically needed to complete various given tasks. Ultimately this approach provided a way in which to account for different performance levels among the staff members without jeopardizing the accuracy of the patient classification system. The data collected from the time-and-motion study indicated that the routine of a bed bath took anywhere from 13 to 18 minutes (Exhibits 11-3 and 11-4). Therefore, with this information taken into consideration a complete bed bath was assigned a relative value unit of 3.

By arbitrarily defining the range of each relative value unit, each nursing task could be assigned a certain RVU, depending on the time and complexity involved in performing the relative task. In cases where the data yielded two RVU ranges, the group elected to average the time involved. For example, the data indicated that foley catheter irrigations required 8 minutes to 15 minutes. What RVU should be assigned: 2 or 3? Adding both ranges (23 minutes) and dividing by 2 yields the average of 11.5. Hence, foley catheter irrigations were assigned a relative value unit of 2. Exhibit 11-5 illustrates the results and final products achieved after compiling all of these efforts.

There are several loopholes in this time-and-motion study. For example, standard treatments (coughing, deep breathing, vital signs every shift, TED stockings, etc.) were omitted. Three to five routine medications or two PRNs per shift took approximately 7 to 12 minutes to dispense. But some patients take three to five routine medications *and* two PRNs per shift. This particular combination of medications had been overlooked in the initial development of the system. Such loopholes were readily identified by the nursing staff throughout the hospital once the system was implemented on a trial basis.

By the staff's own admission this first attempt at developing an objective, differential basis for a patient classification system was anything but a total success story. Frequent repositioning and interruptions such as occasional incontinence of patients may be categorized differently by individual staff members. There was no process to assure patients that they were being cared for by the appropriately trained staff member (RN, LVN, NA).

Exhibit 11-3 Time-and-Motion Study—Model A

$7^{00} \rightarrow 7^{47}$	— arrived late for work
$7^{47} \rightarrow 8^{05}$	√ assignment sheet + get report of Pat's notes
$8^{05} \rightarrow 8^{10}$	start partial bedbath in 105, √ IVAC, √ heparin plug, √ dressing.
$8^{10} \rightarrow 8^{25}$	get report off rand
$8^{25} \rightarrow 8^{45}$	complete 105's bath, ambulate c̄ IVAC to B Station + return to make bed.
$8^{45} \rightarrow 9$	Assist Dr c̄ suture removal + drsg. change.
$9 \rightarrow 9^{05}$	√ on pain med - inform pt. too early
$9^{05} \rightarrow 9^{15}$	Partial bath completed on 104B, discussion about f/c dc + saving urine
$9^{15} \rightarrow 9^{30}$	Sterile drsg chg. 104, ~~be~~ linen chg, √ urine (1st void p̄ f/c dc'd)
$9^{30} \rightarrow 9^{35}$	Ambulate in hallway
$9^{35} \rightarrow 9^{40}$	Put 118 in shower, look for pj pants, found some on C station, give to pt. in shower.
$9^{40} \rightarrow 9^{45}$	Get tub ready for 109A
$9^{45} \rightarrow 9^{50}$	√ IV in 103, medicate 105B
$9^{50} \rightarrow 10^{10}$	Pass 10 o'clock meds

Exhibit 11-3 continued

$10^{10} \rightarrow 10^{15}$	Chg drsg on 118A, medicate 118A
$10^{15} \rightarrow 10^{25}$	Sterile drg chg 101B, set up partial bath.
$10^{25} \rightarrow 10^{30}$	Inform 105 no further narcotics, give comfort
$10^{30} \rightarrow 10^{45}$	Cath care, leg bag change, ambulate 101B in hallway
$10^{45} \rightarrow 10^{50}$	Linen change.
$10^{50} \rightarrow 10^{60}$	√ chart, get B+W for 101B
$11^{01} \rightarrow 11^{02}$	Call pharm re: Hyperal
$11^{03} \rightarrow 11^{10}$	Pick up hyperal, √ 3x5 card c̄ bottle, (call pharm re: hyperlyte) mark label for time, hang bottle, irrigate S Sump.
$11^{10} \rightarrow 11^{15}$	Medicate 109A, √ chart for laxative order
$11^{15} \rightarrow 11^{30}$	Help c̄ alcohol sponge bath in 125A, hang rider (draw up + give NS, clear tubing, tape down + position arm)
$11^{30} \rightarrow 12$	Lunch
$12 \rightarrow 12^{15}$	Chart medications, √ pts., Med. 120B
$12^{15} \rightarrow 12^{30}$	Pass trays, set up pts.
$12^{30} \rightarrow 1$	NCPlans –
$1 \rightarrow 1^{15}$	Insert f/c, √ for outcome, connect to CDU, reassure pt.

Exhibit 11-3 continued

115→120	√105, Reassure, ↑commode + back to bed
120→130	Pass H_2O and juice, Dc IV 103
130→155	Collect I+O's (empty foley, empty leg bags), √ IV totals, ice chips for 105
155→2	Report to Pat
2→240	Chart nurses notes—talk c̄ Dr McCole, NCPlan formulation
240→243	Medicate 118 for HA
245→3	Medicate 124A, get crackers + jc 124B
3	√ medication c̄ pharm (by phone)
305→310	Medicate 118A
310→320	Finish charting
320→330	Get nar + hyp out for count
330→340	Count nar + hyp.

18 May 80

101B	Mar March	(PO day 4)
102A	Angina	(Hosp day 8)
104B	Mar March	(PO day 5)
105B	Gastro-Jeju	(PO day 8)
109A	Sig + Hem	(PO day 3)
118A	Cerv Discect.	(PO day 4)
103B	IV's	

EBoomeren
TPC–6 pts

2nd of 5

Source: Reprinted with permission of Nursing Department, Doctors Hospital of Pinole, Pinole, California.

Exhibit 11-4 Time-and-Motion Study—Model B

9/13/83	assignment: 5 pts total care and meds, IV's and riders for orderly's 5 pts
3 - 3:45	report + get assignment ; take post-op vitals
3:45 - 3:55	check trach + called RT and CS for supplies
3:55 - 4:05	make rounds to assigned pts - ck IV's
4:05 - 4:15	go to CS + get supplies
4:15 - 4:30	review rand for pt care & meds
4:30 - 4:40	bring pt from admitting to room
4:40 - 5:10	pour + pass meds & hang riders
5:10 - 5:25	start to admit pt
5:25 - 5:40	IV rider + get instructions from RT on trach care
5:40 - 5:50	pt care + talk to pt's family + obtain vitals + S & A's
5:50 - 6:00	pass dinner trays
6:00 - 6:10	finish reviewing randcards
6:10 - 6:20	two pain hypos
6:20 - 6:30	finish admitting pt
6:30 - 6:45	IV riders & pass meds
6:45 - 7:00	pt care + ck orders (strain urine, measurements for tx, ck K-pads + dressings)
7:00 - 7:20	ck IV's and do some charting
7:20 - 7:45	pt care (pre-op shower, linen change - pre-op urine)
7:45 - 7:55	pour meds
7:55 - 8:15	pt care (NG irrigation - refill magnacal for NG feedings - ck drsgs + cms - strain urine)
8:15 - 8:40	dinner break
8:40 - 9:00	begin pm care (vitals, backrubs, fresh water, empty waste baskets)
9:00 - 9:15	pain meds - call supervisor for meds from pharmacy - take sups to pharm
9:15 - 9:45	continue pm care + vitals
9:45 - 10:15	start to pass 10:00 meds + riders
10:15 - 10:25	IV infiltrated - d'cd
10:25 - 10:55	finish passing meds & riders . (heparinize plugs)

Exhibit 11-4 continued

10:45 - 10:55	get I + Os · empty Foley
10:55 - 11:05	give report to head nurse
11:05 - 11:20	pt pulled out NG tube - complete linen change (magnacal all over bed)
11:20 – 11:30	go to C.S. for new NG tube
11:30 - 11:50	reinsert NG
11:50 – 12:00	complete IV board + additional report to night shift
12:00 – 1:00	charting

(whew!)

Source: Reprinted with permission of Nursing Department, Doctors Hospital of Pinole, Pinole, California.

Despite the loopholes, the nursing staff was committed to perfecting a workable system. Week after week the unit coordinators and charge nurses continued to meet, attempting to revise the system based on written input and suggestions from the nursing staff. These suggestions were infinite and for the most part repetitious. However, one thought-provoking suggestion—why not have the patient classification system parallel the kardex?—soon became a reality. While once again another form (Exhibit 11-5) met its demise, its successor (Exhibit 11-6) emerged.

FUNDAMENTAL SKILL LEVELS

The patient classification system presented in Exhibit 11-6 was far more objective than any of its predecessors. It definitely defined patient activities in relation to skill level. Ambulation and repositioning activities can be managed by all staff members, but oral medications may be dispensed only by RNs and LVNs. The relative value unit is assigned to the most fundamental skill level required to carry out the activity. Therefore, in the case of ambulation the RVU is assigned to the NA column, while in the case of oral medication administration the RVU is assigned to the LVN column. In this way, patient activities are carried out according to the skill level required rather than according to room number or proximity to the nurses' station. The columns of activities were added according to skill level, totaled, dated, and initialed by the individual designated responsible for the assessment process.

To examine the effectiveness of this particular patient classification system, let us consider a hypothetical situation. James Gordon is a 50-year-old male admitted

Exhibit 11-5 Patient Acuity System Guidelines—Model A

	MEDICATIONS		I.Vs.		TREATMENTS
					(IF TREATMENT IS COMPLEX + 1 PT.)
1	2 ROUTINE MEDS OR 1 PRN PER SHIFT.	1	TKO - I.Vs TELEMETRY HEP. PLUG	1	MINIMAL BEDSIDE CARE, S & A, DAILY STANDING WEIGHTS, K-PAD ICE COLLARS.
2	3 - 5 ROUTINE MEDS OR 2 PRNs PER SHIFT.	2	q 8 HRS. IVPB'S OR PUSHES 8, 10, 12 HRS. IV's	2	AM. CATH CARE, ENEMA, I & O, COMPRESSES & DOUCH, DRESSINGS, CATHETERIZATION & PRE-OP PREPS, VITALS q 4 HRS. NURO q 4 HRS.
3	6 - 10 ROUTINE MEDS OR 3 TO 4 PRNs PER SHIFT.	3	q 4 HRS. & 6 HRS. IVPB's AND PUSH RAPID RATE IV's.	3	DECUBITIS CARE, COLOSTOMY CARE, TELEMETRY.
4	11 OR MORE ROUTINE MEDS OR MORE THAN 5 PRNs PER SHIFT.	4	TPN, TRANFUSIONS COMPLEX I.V. PUSHES.	4	SUCTIONING, WOUND IRRIGATIONS.
		5	HEP. INFUSION, PLATELETS FREQUENCY 1,2,3 HRS. IVPB's 2 OR MORE I.V. SITES AT ONCE.		
	ACTIVITY		**EXCRETION**		**GROOMING**
1	AMBULATORY	1	SELF CARE	1	SELF CARE
2	AMB. OR TURN WITH HELP	2	REQUIRES ASSISTANCE (1)	2	BED BATH WITH HELP
3	AMB. OR TURN WITH HELP(2 NURSES)	3	REQUIRES ASSISTANCE (2) OR OCCASIONAL INCONTINENCE	3	COMPLETE CARE - ALERT PATIENT
4	FREQUENT REPOSITIONING ROM, ETC.	4	INCONTENENCE (MORE THAN TWICE PER SHIFT)	4	COMPLETE CARE WITH COMATOSE PT. OR PT. WITH COMPLICATED EQUIPMENT.

ADDED SPECIAL CONDITIONS/PROCEDURES:________________ TOTAL DAILY ACUITY:________

ROOM:______ NAME: ____________ DIAGNOSIS:____________ AGE:______ DOCTOR:________

Exhibit 11-5 continued

	BEHAVIOR		TEACHING	
1	ALERT - ORIENTED	1	ROUTINE	
2	MILDLY CONFUSED; DEPRESSED (RESTRAIN FOR SAFETY)	2	RE-INFORCEMENT	
3	VERY CONFUSED; DEPRESSED	3	NEW DIAGNOSIS (REQUIRES COMPLETE TEACHING)	
4	AGITATED, DEMANDING, D.T'S	4	COMPLETE TEACHING PROBLEMS e.g.(COMMUNICATION BARRIERS)	

ADDED SPECIAL CONDITIONS/PROCEDURES:____________ TOTAL DAILY ACUITY:________

ROOM: ____ NAME:________ DIAGNOSIS:________ AGE:____ DOCTOR:________

Source: Reprinted with permission of Nursing Department, Doctors Hospital of Pinole, Pinole, California.

to the hospital on August 25, 1983. For six weeks before admission he has suffered intermittent right upper-quadrant pain, always most severe after the ingestion of a fatty meal. He seeks the expertise of his internist, who has Mr. Gordon undergo various testing procedures. The definitive diagnosis is cholecystitis; the recommended treatment is surgical intervention: cholecystectomy. This is Mr. Gordon's first encounter with illness requiring hospitalization; he had always been healthy and required no routine medications. On August 26, 1983, a cholecystectomy is performed. Mr. Gordon returns to the postoperative unit with an IV infusing into his right hand, a large dressing covering the incision, and a nasogastric tube in place. The physician's orders are as follows:

- Patient NPO.
- Vital signs q4h around the clock.
- Change abdominal dressing q shift and prn—patient has penrose drain in incision.
- Dangle this P.M. and progessive ambulation in A.M.
- Turn, cough, and deep breathe q2h while awake.
- TED hose.
- Irrigate NG tube q shift and prn.
- Follow present IV with 1,000 cc D5 1/2NS with 20 mEq KCl at 125 cc per hour.
- Meds:
  —Keflin Gm. 1 IVPB q6h
  —Demerol 100 mg and Vistaril 50 mg IM q3-4h prn pain
  —Seconal 100 mg IM prn sleep
- CBC, electrolytes in A.M.

The physician's orders are incorporated into Mr. Gordon's care plan, which appears in Exhibit 11-7. Referring to Exhibit 11-7, the reader can correlate the information documented on the care plan with the patient classification system (Exhibit 11-6). Some activities are absolutes, so to speak, and the nursing staff can remain 100 percent objective. Vital signs every 4 hours, routine dressing changes, intake and output, and NPO are examples of such absolutes, which leave no room for varying interpretations.

However, some areas of patient care do require some subjective evaluations on the part of the nursing staff. For example, prn medications require projected nursing judgments. Here the nursing staff has indicated that Mr. Gordon will require 4 to 6 prn medications over the next 24 hours. Since the physician has ordered pain medication every 3 to 4 hours, Mr. Gordon could conceivably receive six to eight injections in the following 24 hours.

Exhibit 11-6 Patient Acuity System Guidelines—Model B

TREATMENTS	RN	LVN	NA
	acuity units		
Hemovac		1	
Sugar & Acetest			1
Ice collar			1
Standing weights			1
Douche		1	
Cath care			1
Vital signs q shift			1
Hemastix			1
Strain urine			1
C, T, D.B.			1
Specimen collection			1
K-pad			1
Back rub			1
Routine dressing changes		1	
Oxygen		1	
Oral suction		1	
I & O			2
Bedscale weights			2
Enemas			2
VS q 4 hours			2
Sterile compresses		2	
Routine traction		2	
Foley irrigations		2	
Straight or Foley cath.		2	
Skeletal traction		2	
Chest tubes		2	
NG Tubes/Irrigation		2	

	RN	LVN	NA
	acuity units		
Starting IV or changing heparin plug	2		
VS q 2-3 hours			3
Pre-op Shaves & Preps		3	
Complicated dressing changes	3		
Decubitus care		3	
Colostomy/Ileal care		3	
Telemetry		3	
Difficult IV	3		
VS and/or NS q 1 hour		4	
Nasal/Trach suctioning		4	
Trach care		4	
Subclavian Dressing	4		
Neuros. q 4 hours		2	
Neuros. q 2-3 hours		3	
GROOMING			
Self-care			1
Bed bath w/ help			2
Complete care w/ cooperative pt.			3
Complete care w/ comatose pt., difficult pt., and/or complicated equipment		4	
ACTIVITY			
Ambulatory; BRP			0
Ambulate and/or turn w/ help; Bedrest			2
Ambulate (2 nurses required):			
Difficult patient to turn			3
Frequent repositioning; ROM			4

	acuity units		
	RN	LVN	NA
EXCRETION			
Self-care			0
Requires assistance			1
Requires assistance (2 nurses)			3
Occasional incontinence; Frequest trips to BR			4
Incontinence (more than twice/shift)			5
BEHAVIOR			
Alert & oriented			0
Mildly confused; depressed			2
Very confused, depressed, or anxious pt.			3
Agitated, demanding, constant supervision and/ or restraints			6
TEACHING: PATIENT OR FAMILY			
Routine		1	
Reinforcement, pre-op teaching		2	
New diagnosis, requires complete teaching	3		
Repeated instruction and/or demonstrations w/ patient or family	4		
FEEDING			
NPO or feeds self			1
Needs preparation, food cut, tray set up			2
Feeder, push fluids, fluid restriction			3
Difficult feeder, NG feedings w/ suctioning; calorie count		4	
NG feedings & difficult feeder		7	

	acuity units		
	RN	LVN	NA
ISOLATION			
Respiratory		3	
Enteric		3	
Wound and Skin		4	
Strict		7	
ROUTINE MEDICATIONS: PO, IM, OR SQ			
1-3 meds per day		1	
4-6 meds per day		2	
7-10 meds per day		3	
11-13 meds per day		4	
Greater than 13, add one point for each three additional meds		*	
PRN MEDICATIONS			
1-3 prns per day		1	
4-6 prns per day		2	
7-10 prns per day		3	
11-13 prns per day		4	
Greater than 13, add one point for each three additional prns		*	
IVs			
Heparin plug w/ daily irrigation	1		
Cont. IVs (TKO, q8, q10, or q12)	2		
Cont. IVs (q4, q6)	3		

Exhibit 11-6 continued

	acuity units		
	RN	LVN	NA
MEDICATIONS VIA CONTINUOUS IV			
1-3 meds per day	(1)		
4-6 meds per day	2		
7-10 meds per day	3		
11-13 meds per day	4		
IV MEDS VIA HEPARIN PLUG OR COMPLICATED IV			
IV med × 1 per shift	3		
IV med × 2 per shift	4		
IV med × 3 per shift	5		
IVAC MEDS (TPN, Heparin, Aminophylline, FFP, Platelets, Chemotherapy)	6		
Blood Transfusions	6		

RN	LVN	NA	TOTAL ACUITY
4	6	13	23

LOG

DAY	DATE	ACUITY	NURSE
1	8/26	23	PAC
2			
3			
4			
5			
6			
7			

Gordon, James
PATIENT'S NAME

Source: Reprinted with permission of Nursing Department, Doctors Hospital of Pinole, Pinole, California.

Exhibit 11-7 Patient Care Plan

DOCTORS HOSPITAL - PINOLE **PATIENT CARE PLAN**

CODE STATUS

ISOLATION:

ALLERGIES: ND KNOWN ALLERGIES

BRIEF MEDICAL HISTORY: FIRST HOSPITALIZATION

DISCHARGE PLANS:

NURSING DX/PROBLEM	GOAL (LONG & SHORT TERM)	NURSING ACTION
Immobility	Pt able to ambulate s̄ assistance by 8/28	Dangle pm 8/25; Chair by 7Am 8/26
		Ambulate in room c̄ help 10A 2p 8/26
		Ambulate in hall c̄ help 6p 9p 8/26
		Ambulate in hall c̄ help QID 8/27
		Ambulate in hall s̄ help QID 8/28

ADM. DATE	TO ICU/CCU	TO FLOOR	RELIGION	HOSP. NO.
8/25			BAPT	01234

ADM. DX: Cholecystitis

CURRENT DX:

SURG. DATE	SURGICAL PROCEDURE	DATE	SPECIAL PROCEDURES
8/26	Cholecystectomy		

DIET: 8/26 NPO

Assist c̄ Tray

Feed

Tube Feedings

Fluids:

Exhibit 11-7 continued

	DATE	
BATH		Shower/Tub
		Partial
	X	Complete 8/26
		Sitz Bath
OBSERVATIONS		Weight Bedscale Bathscale
	X	TPR 2A 6A 10A 2p 6p 10p
	X	BP
		Neuro Checks
		Pedal Pulse Check
		Cast and CMST Check
	X	I & O D.O. Last BM
	X	Dressing Check Change 6A 2p 10p and prn
		Compresses
		K Pad
MOBILITY		Bedrest X Dangle prn 8/25
	X	Chair 8/26
	X	BRP 8/26 Help [X]
	X	Ambulate qid 8/26 Help [X]
		Turn & Position
		Active/Passive ROM
		Leg Exercises
		Physical Therapy:

	DATE	
VENT	X	Cough & Deep Breath q 2° while awake
		Cont. Mech. Aide Vent.
		Oral & Nasal Suctioning
		Oxygen
		Resp. Therapy
TREATMENTS		Clinitest and Acetest
		Colostomy Irrigation and Care
		Decubitus Care
		Eggshell Mattress
		Foot Cradle
		Overhead Frame & Trapeze
		Restraints
		Sheepskin
	X	Teds 8/25
		Telemetry/Monitor
		Trach Care
		Traction

ACUITY ASSESSMENT

Physical					
Medication/Treatments					
Observation					
Psycho./Social					
Instructional					

Date: ________

Nurse: ________

	DATE	
TUBES		Foley Catheter
		Cath. Care
		Irrigate Foley
		Clamp Foley
		Cath. Change [ ]
		Cath. Dc'd [ ] → Check
		Time & Amount of Each Voiding
		Chest Tube
		Chest Tube Milking
		Chest Tube Dc'd [ ]
		Hemovac
		Jackson Pratt
	X	NG Tube Irrigate 6A 2p 10p and prn
		Irrigate Ng Tube
		Ng Tube Dc'd [ ]
		Penrose Drain Dc'd [ ]
		Shunt
		Sutures Dc'd [ ]
LINES		H. P. Insert [ ]
		H. P. Change Due [ ]
	X	IV Insert [8/25]
	X	IV Change Due [8/27]
		Other Lines:
	X	IV: 1000 cc D5 ½ NS c̄ 20 mEq KCl at 125cc/hour

BEGIN	ROUTINE MEDS	TIME	DC
8/26	Keflin ī gram IVPB q6°	5-11-5-11	8/30

BEGIN	PRN MEDICATIONS	TIME	DC
8/26	Demerol 100mg, Vistaril 50mg IM q3-4° prn pain		8/30

	H S MEDS		
8/26	Seconal 100mg IM prn sleep		8/30

DATE	LAB
8/26	CBC Electrolytes 8/27

DATE	X-RAY

DATE	NUCLEAR MEDICINE

RELATIVE & PHONE NUMBER: Mrs. Jennifer Gordon (513) 277-8160

CONSULTING PHYSICIAN:

ROOM: 634 | NAME M.S. D.W.: JAMES GORDON | AGE: 60 | PRIMARY PHYSICIAN: DOCTOR ROBERT MURRAY

FORM DH 505-07

Source: Reprinted with permission of Doctors Hospital of Pinole, Pinole, California.

Several factors will be considered before the nursing staff can reasonably decide how much pain medication is necessary to keep Mr. Gordon comfortable. Mr. Gordon's preoperative state of mind will be assessed. Is he alert and cooperative? Is he afraid of pain? Is he extremely anxious? His height and weight will also be considered in relation to the amount of medication ordered by the physician. Does the amount ordered correspond with his height and weight as recommended in the literature? Does the pain medication include an analgesic potentiator? What routine medications are ordered (muscle relaxers, sedatives, tranquilizers)? Finally, past experience with postoperative patients will influence the decision made by the nursing staff. How many pain injections does the average postoperative cholecystectomy patient require?

After considering such factors, the nursing staff must make a subjective projection. The nursing staff finds Mr. Gordon alert, cooperative, and free from excessive anxiety. His pain medication includes an analgesic potentiator; the dosages correspond with his height and weight. Past experience indicated that postoperative patients generally require four to six pain injections the first 24 hours following surgery. For these reasons the nursing staff projects that Mr. Gordon probably requires four to six pain injections.

Both the objective activities and the subjective projections provide the nursing staff with Mr. Gordon's total acuity (23) as well as the acuity according to skill level (RN = 4, LVN = 6, NA = 13). The total patient acuity represents the greatest amount of time expressed in RVUs expended in 24 hours to care for a patient as defined by the patient classification system. By utilizing basic mathematical equations, one can determine both the minimum and the maximum amount of nursing time expended on the care of Mr. Gordon per shift. (One RVU is assigned to an activity requiring less than 6 minutes to perform.)

If one RVU is assigned to an activity requiring less than 6 minutes to perform, then the minimum time required for one RVU activity is 1 minute; the maximum time is by definition 6 minutes. Therefore, if Mr. Gordon has been assigned an acuity of 23 (X = 23 RVU), the minimum amount of time required would be 1 minute per RVU or

$$X = 23 \text{ RVU}$$

and a minimum RVU equals 1 minute:

$$X \text{ minimum} = 23 \text{ minutes}$$

Similarly the maximum amount of time required would be 6 minutes per RVU or

$$X = 23 \text{ RVU}$$

and maximum RVU equals 6 minutes:

$$X = 23 \times 6 \text{ minutes} =$$
$$138 \text{ minutes} = 2 \text{ hours, } 18 \text{ minutes}$$

One can also determine the minimum and maximum amount of nursing time expended according to skill level by using the same mathematical process. The following figures are representative of that process.

Skill Level	*Minimum Time/Shift*	*Maximum Time/Shift*
RN	4 minutes	24 minutes
LVN	6 minutes	36 minutes
NA	13 minutes	78 minutes (1 hour, 18 minutes)

Of course, as Mr. Gordon's condition improves from day to day, the amount of nursing time expended will decrease accordingly.

PATIENT ASSIGNMENT

Not only did this particular patient classification system allow a differentiation of patient care according to skill level; it also provided a way in which to distribute patient assignments evenly. Consider the following patients and their acuity levels.

Patient	*Room #*	*RN*	*LVN*	*NA*	*Total*
Rick Smith	633	4	6	12	22
Mary Black	637	2	6	10	18
Gary Jones	638	0	0	10	10
Nancy White	642	2	0	8	10
Ruth Little	643	4	0	6	10
Kevin Brown	644	0	0	6	6
	Total	12	12	52	76

Three staff members are available to care for these patients: Kathy Miller, RN; Joan Rider, LVN; and Martha Reed, NA. If RN Miller were to care for all 6 patients alone, her total assignment would equal 76 RVUs. If LVN Rider were to assume the same patient assignment, the acuity would equal 64 (52 + 12 RVUs), while RN Miller would assume the remaining 12 RVUs. For the most part, most RVUs assumed by the RN would be those related to IV therapy. Hence, those RVUs are labeled as IVs on the daily patient assignment form. Typical patient assignments appear in Exhibit 11-2.

This method of patient assignment improved distribution of patient care and staff morale. For once, quality nursing care was delivered according to skill level. In fact, the patient classification system paralleled the job descriptions in terms of technical skills and patient activities. It was virtually impossible to request and allow individuals to perform any nursing activity for which they were not qualified. Everything was written in black and white, delineating clear-cut boundaries between the various different skill levels. Furthermore, complaints about unfair assignments ceased. One's attention was drawn to RVUs as opposed to the number of patients. It became obvious that assigning an equal number of patients to each care giver did not assure equal distribution of patient care. Comments such as "I have 7 patients and Mary only has 6 patients" decreased. Friction between licensed and unlicensed personnel also decreased as patient assignments were more evenly distributed according to acuity. In short this particular patient classification system provided both the nursing administration and the nursing staff a way in which to assess accurately each patient's needs and then distribute patient care accordingly.

On an ongoing basis the nursing staff continued to evaluate, review, and revise the patient classification system. Their success in developing an applicable, realistic differential patient classification system provided further incentive to maintain such a system. Technology and change were beyond their control, but their ability to adapt was not. Vacated unlicensed positions were eventually changed to licensed positions. LVNs/LPNs were encouraged to become certified in intravenous therapy. As these changes evolved, the measurable differences between skill levels became marginal. Because these differences were marginal, allowing for a more harmonious relationship between RNs and LVNs, eventually the nursing staff elected to forego a patient classification system designed to delineate between skill levels. Instead, the patient classification system was once again revised, as illustrated in Exhibit 11-8. Omitting skill levels was not the only revision. Critical care drugs requiring special monitoring devices as well as sophisticated x-ray and laboratory procedures requiring nursing time were incorporated in the latest patient classification system. The final, and perhaps the most significant, addition was the step that actually integrated the patient classification system with the kardex. Including the patient classification system in this manner has proved a time-saving mechanism for the nursing staff.

Developing and implementing a time-saving device often requires time-consuming activities. For example, the more objective the patient classification system is, the more time-consuming the process of developing the system. The more objective the system is, the more time-consuming the process of assessing patients. The more objective the system is, the more time-consuming the process of reviewing and revising the system. However, the more objective the system is, the less time-consuming the process of accounting for nursing productivity to the financial administrator. Nursing administrators cannot develop and implement

Exhibit 11-8 Patient Care Plan

DOCTORS HOSPITAL - PINOLE

PATIENT CARE PLAN

CODE STATUS

ISOLATION:

ALLERGIES:

BRIEF MEDICAL HISTORY:

DISCHARGE PLANS:

DATE	DX/PROBLEM	GOAL (LONG & SHORT TERM)	ACTION

ADM. DATE		TO ICU/CCU	TO FLOOR	RELIGION	HOSP. NO.

ADM. DX:

CURRENT DX:

DIET:

SURG. DATE	SURGICAL PROCEDURE	DATE	SPECIAL PROCEDURES

Assist c̄ Tray

Feed

Tube Feedings

Fluids:

Exhibit 11-8 continued

	DATE		ACUITY ASSESSMENT
BATH		1	Sitz Bath
		1	Self Care / Shower / Tub
		2	Partial Bath
		3	Complete Bed Bath
		5	Complete Bed Bath w/Diff. Pt.
		1	Shampoo
DIET		1	NPO / Feeds Self
		2	Assist. w/Tray
		3	Feed Patient
		4	Difficult Feeder or Tube Feeding
		5	Keofeed
		7	Difficult Feeder and Tube Feeding
MOBILITY		0	Amublatory / B.R.P.
		1	Dangle
		2	Active / Passive R.O.M.
		2	B.P.R. w/Help X per Shift
		2	Chair w/Help X per Shift
		2	Commode w/Help X per Shift
		3	Ambulate w/Help
		3	Bedrest/Turn & Position Q 2H
MONITOR		1	Cast & C.S.M.T. Check/Pulse Check
		1	Weight · Bathscale ☐ or Bedscale ☐
			Neuro Check Q ____
			T.P.R. · B.P. Q ____
			(Give one pt. for each V.S. or N.S. Check/Shift)
		1	Telemetry / Monitor
NEUR		0	Comatose
		1	Restrain
		2	Confused – Noncombative
		5	Confused – Combative
VENT.		1	Chest Tube (DC'D /)
		1	Oxygen
		1	Cough and Deep Breath
		2	Oral Suctioning
		2	Chest Tube / Emerson Pump
		3	Nasopharyngeal Suctioning
		4	Trach Suctioning and Care
		5	Respirator
OTHER		0	K Pad
		1	Foot Cradle
		1	Overhead Frame
		0	Sheepskin
		1	Egg Crate Mattress
		1	TEDS
		2	Hypothermia Blanket
		1	Ice Collar
		1	Voice Rest

	DATE		ACUTIY ASSESSMENT
G.I.		1	N. G. Suction
		1	N. G. Irrigation (Routine)
		1	Stool Specimen
		2	Colostomy / Ileal Care
		3	Enemas Till Clear
		6	N. G. Lavage (Active Bleed)
URINARY		0	Foley Catheter: Cath (DC'D /). Check time and amount of each voiding until (/).
		1	Strain Urine
		2	S. & A. Q ____
		1	Hemastix
		1	Quantitive Urine Collection
		1	Foley Care
		1	T.U.R. Foley Irrigation
		1	Clamp Foley
		2	Catheter to be Changed (/)
		2	Straight Catheterization
		2	I. & O.
		3	I. and O. 2H or Greater
			Incont. ( ) times/shift. Give 2 per incont.
		3	Cont. Bladder Irrigation
DRESSING		1	Simple Dressing Change
		1	Sterile Compress
		1	Reinforce Dressing or Check Q H
		2	Simple Decubitus Care
		3	Complex Dressing Change
		4	Subclavian / Swan Ganz Drsng Change
		5	Complex Decubitus Care
TEACH		3	Teaching Home Care, Discharge Planning (10 · 25 min. / Shift)
		7	Emotional Needs / Family Problems (1/2 · 1 hr. / Shift)
		9	Intensive Teaching (– 1 hr. / Shift)
DRAIN		0	Clips / Sutures (DC'D /)
		0	Penrose Drian (DC'D /)
		1	Hemovac (DC'D /)
		1	Jackson Pratt (DC'D /)
		1	X-Ray Procedure
		1	Nuclear Med. Procedure
		1	Cardiology Procedure
TRA.		3	Traction
P.T.		0	Physical Therapy

	DATE		ACUITY ASSESSMENT
ISOLA.		3	Respiratory
		3	Enteric
		4	Wound & Skin
		7	Strict / Reverse
LINES		2	Arterial Line
		2	T. P. N.
		2	A. V. Shunt
		4	Swan Ganz
		4	Cardiac Output
		5	I. C. P.
I.V. MEDS.		3	Lidocaine
		3	Heparin
		3	Aminophylline
		3	Blood Products
		3	Chemo Therapy
		2	IVAC c̄ KCL
I.V. MEDS		5	Dopamine
		5	Nipride
		5	Isuprel
		5	Aramine
SITE		0	H. P. Inserted
		2	H. P. Change Due /
		0	I. V. Inserted
		2	I. V. Change Due /
MEDS		1	1 · 3 / Shift (Includes PRN)
		2	4 · 6 / Shift
		3	7 · 9 / Shift
		4	10 or more / Shift
IVS		2	Cont. I. V. Observation
		1	Change 1 Bottle / Shift
			___ Piggyback/Shift. One pt. per Piggyback/Shift
		2	1 · 3 I.V. Push Meds / Shift
		3	4 · 6 I.V. Push Meds / Shift
R.T.		0	Respiratory Therapy

DATE	ACUITY
SIGNATURE	

BEGIN	ROUTINE MEDS	TIME	DC	BEGIN	PRN MEDICATIONS	TIME	DC
					H S MEDS		
				DATE	LAB		
				DATE	X-RAY		
				DATE	NUCLEAR MEDICINE		

RELATIVE & PHONE NUMBER			CONSULTING PHYSICIAN
ROOM	NAME M.S. D.W.	AGE	PRIMARY PHYSICIAN FORM DH 505-07

Source: Reprinted with permission of Doctors Hospital of Pinole, Pinole, California.

effective systems alone. They must encourage and continue to encourage input and suggestions from the grass-roots level, namely, the nursing staff.

With this system the nursing administrator will be prepared to document estimates each time the financial administrator seeks justification for nursing hours. The staffing system was developed carefully and objectively to provide for delivery of the quality of care that nursing mandated, the quality of care that the physicians practiced, and the quality of care that the patient warranted. The effective nursing administrator will continue to encourage the nursing staff to update the patient classification system. It should not be allowed to become dormant, for it is the only method of justifying time, hours, and productivity.

Chapter 12

Staffing by Tradition or Staffing by Policy? The Importance of Developing Structured Staffing Policy

OBJECTIVES

Following completion of this chapter the reader will be able to:

- list the five basic components of successful management,
- list the three criteria that should be considered when developing staffing policy, and
- list the five staffing policy topics that should be present in any nursing department.

During the early 1900s the first steps in a systematic approach to management were taken by Frederick W. Taylor, an engineer in the steel industry. Before Taylor's research into scientific management, most management decisions had been made on the basis of a supervisor's experience in handling related problems. Managers frequently had limited knowledge of how to deal with problems. The traditional attitude of "but we've always done it that way" was the rationale used for dealing with many employee problems.[1]

Since 1900 management has become progressively more aware of the human elements: that people are not machines and that principles of management must take into account these human elements. The success or failure of a nursing department, or any business, to a great extent relies on the attitudes and motivation of the people forming its cornerstone structures. It is the responsibility of the department managers to motivate individuals to ensure achievable success.

Five basic components of successful management are generally recognized and accepted in the management world. They are:

1. planning,
2. organizing,

3. directing,
4. coordinating, and
5. controlling.[2]

These five basic components must be considered when a manager establishes any new protocol in a department; the human element must be included in each component.[3]

Developing a structured staffing policy is part of the controlling component essential to successful management. The reasons for this have become clear-cut and universally accepted by all members of the nursing department. First, everyone needs rules, limits, and boundaries; nurses are by no means an exception to the rule. Ideally the rules and limits should parallel the staffing guidelines. Second, an even more sound reason for developing specific staffing policies is to provide the proper patient/nurse ratios as recommended by JCAH, various state codes, and each individual institution's standards of practice. A written staffing policy spells out policies in black and white, accomplishes described standards, and leaves less room for misinterpreting the policy or manipulating the staffing system. Third, good staffing policies result in improved morale and evidence of a team spirit, as everyone with access to the policy electively chooses to follow it.

TRADITIONAL STAFFING

In many hospitals nurse staffing has randomly been accomplished through traditional modes. Frequently the staffing guidelines are more or less mandated by the employees or by outdated practices. Many of the traditional staffing policies are based on past staffing procedures or the subjectivity of the supervisors or staffing coordinators. It is only human nature that if no policy exists—no rules or limits or boundaries—then the system can be and often is manipulated at will. The mechanism for staffing any particular unit may be decided because it has always been done that way. Yet little in the volumes of nursing department policy manuals supports the traditional staffing policies in many hospitals.

Staffing policy and staffing guidelines in many institutions are often fragmented, inconsistent, and individualized according to the employees' needs rather than the benefit of management's rules and needs. While the individual employee who may benefit from the lack of structured staffing policy may be happy, the result and untoward effect on other department employees can be less than pleasant particularly when it results in confusing schedules, excessively long work stretches, unfair holiday work schedules, and a label of favoritism being attached to the nursing administration.

Chapter 1 deals with the need, from a nursing administration standpoint, for limits, controls, and documentation as set by JCAH standards and the state of

California's Title 22. While staff nurses need staffing policies detailed and spelled out, so management needs staffing policies detailed and spelled out.

In the past, nursing managers have been barraged with language about the nursing shortage, nursing burnout, and the large number of nurses desiring to leave the profession for total career change. Staff nurses talked about needing a greater challenge in their careers. Because of this, nursing management has been scared into believing that it must develop staffing policies according to what the employee needs and desires instead of what management and the facility may need and desire for delivering the quality of care described in its standards.

Another common problem is that many nursing managers, that is, unit coordinators (head nurses) and department supervisors, do not fully understand the working concept of position control. There frequently is little awareness within the personnel department of the nursing department's precise staffing needs as they relate to position control. (See Chapter 14 for a discussion of position control.) As a result, a great deal of passing of the buck can occur when no one will admit to the problems associated with position control or rather the lack of position control and staffing control. In institutions where a staffing system and position control are in place, the nursing administration needs to communicate with the personnel department of the hospital so that questions and concerns relating to personnel matters can be properly answered.

CRITERIA FOR EFFECTIVE STAFFING

A number of criteria must be present when one is developing an effective staffing policy. Important features to consider are the following:

- A staffing policy must be developed that is unique to the particular institution for which it will serve. Any labor agreements and professional nursing contract agreements must be considered. If flexible staffing or 12-hour shifts are a desired outcome, the staffing policy must allow for continuity of care and the ability to achieve departmental and unit goals, as well as allowing for the philosophy of the staffing system itself to grow and flourish.
- Nursing administration should research scheduling alternatives to determine the feasibility and the anticipated costs involved for the specific staffing policy.
- A realistic policy must be created by the nursing administrative middle management group, that is, assistant directors, supervisors, unit coordinators, or head nurses, but should be reviewed and approved by the nursing administrator. When finalized, the nursing administrative middle management group should then design methods to implement the policy process.

It is highly recommended that the following staffing policies exist in all nursing departments. Additional policies should deal with the individual needs of specialty departments and the overall facility.

Allocation of Personnel

A policy in the nursing administration should describe how registered nurses and licensed vocational nurses (or licensed practical nurses) will be allocated. This allocation should occur according to patient care needs. As patient census and acuity fluctuate, so do the *number* and *type* of personnel needed to deliver quality patient care. Since a minimum number of registered nurses will be needed on a nursing unit, in spite of patient acuity or patient census, a nursing administration should develop guidelines to justify a specific RN/LVN ratio. This justification will be used for patient acuity.

Determining Staffing Requirements

A necessary policy states that staffing requirements will be based on the assessment of patient needs considering, but not limited to, the following:

- ability of the patient to care for self
- the degree of the illness of the patient
- any requirements for special nursing activities
- the skill level of personnel required to do patient care
- the placement of the patient on the nursing unit

Assigning Nursing Care of Patients to Nursing Staff

A policy should specify how the assignment of patients to nursing personnel is determined. The policy should also show how this decision is reached. For example, the policy might state: The unit coordinator or charge nurse on each shift will make assignments of patient care giving consideration to the qualifications of the individual assigned to give that care as well as the needs of the patient.

The Use of a Float Staff

A written policy should address utilization of the "float" staff. In other words, how is it decided which members of the nursing staff have flexible/cross-trained qualifications and can work in other nursing units by floating from med/surg to the emergency department, critical care or outpatient units when the need arises? To adjust to the fluctuations in workloads on nursing units, nursing staff should be appropriately reassigned, instead of resorting to calling in additional staff.

If a per-diem staff or full-time/part-time float pool is developed, these members should be capable of supplementing regular staff when necessary. Some hospitals operate successfully by using a float pool of nursing personnel who are not assigned to a specific unit on a predetermined basis but rather assigned to a nursing unit dependent on fluctuations in patient acuity levels, unit census, and staffing shortages related to sick calls, etc.

Assignment of Registry Personnel

Registry personnel or contract personnel are those nursing personnel employed by an outside agency that contracts with a hospital (or other health care facility) to provide temporary nursing care services. The cost is higher than normally paid to hospital-employed nursing personnel. Nursing administrations should insist that any outside agency with whom they contract have a mechanism to verify current state licensure, past employee records, as well as a mechanism for periodical performance review from all hospitals where the registry employee has worked. Further, each hospital should create written criteria describing how registry nurses are to be utilized within the nursing department. An example of such a policy might be, if a registry nurse reports to duty without a proper written evaluation from the contracting agency before working in the hospital, the placement of that nurse shall be limited to those nursing care units that are supervised by an experienced RN who is a regular member of the hospital nursing staff.

Each nursing department should refer to its state administrative codes for further determination of needed staffing policy. For example, in the state of California, the Administrative Code, Title 22, Division 5, Article 3, Section 70213, states:

> (G) There shall be documentation of the methodology used in making staffing determinations. Such documentations shall be part of the records of the nursing services and be available for review.
>
> (H) There shall be a written staffing pattern which shall show:
> 1. Total numbers of staff, including full-time and full-time equivalents.
> 2. The available nursing care hours for each nursing unit.
> 3. The categories of staff available for patient care.
>
> (I) There shall be a record retained for six months of the written staffing pattern available for review by the department at any given time.

The development of such written guidelines and policies will only enhance the success of staffing patterns. And success among nursing management groups will depend upon their understanding of and ability to implement written guidelines and policies. With adequate planning and organizing, traditional staffing mechanisms can be adapted and converted into more structured, measurable staffing policies. The result will be direct control in allocating personnel to appropriate work assignments. Ultimately the coordination of specific criteria provides the patient with the added benefit of quality care on a consistent basis.

NOTES

1. Dale Carnegie and Associates, *Managing through People* (New York: Simon and Schuster, 1978), p. 15.
2. Ibid., p. 18.
3. A textbook, *Psychology and Contemporary Affairs,* by Nathaniel J. Ehrlich (Monterey, Calif.: Brooks/Cole Publishing Company, 1972) can be a valuable resource to the reader who desires to learn more about a variety of management techniques and experiments used to better understand psychology in the marketplace today. The reader can find in this text descriptions of experiments conducted to show the relationship between increased productivity and employee satisfaction.

Chapter 13

Using a Patient Classification System to Develop a Staffing System

OBJECTIVES

Following completion of this chapter the reader will be able to:

- list five criteria essential for a functioning and effective staffing system,
- describe how a method of justification should be used in a staffing system, and
- state two reasons for documenting positive or negative variances in daily nursing care hours.

A nurse staffing system can be defined as a systematic method of assignment of patients to nursing personnel relating the ability and qualifications of the professional nurse to the degree of illness and needs of the patient as determined from an established patient classification system.[1] As stated in Chapter 8, a staffing system that is reliable, objective, flexible, and universally interpretable must exist in a nursing department. After a carefully thought-out patient classification system has been designed, a nursing department can utilize this system as the major tool for effective nurse staffing. Just as there are wide varieties of patient classification systems, numerous methods are available to staff nursing departments once these patient classification systems are designed.

Principles of nurse staffing are as complex as the individuals who develop and implement them. Like the great matrix of a large corporation, principles of staffing systems are pyramided on one another. The substructure principles of staffing systems are the nuts and bolts of the system itself; the thoroughness with which these principles are thought out and researched will certainly affect the solidity or failure of the system. Just as the short-term goals of the large corporation cannot be met without the understanding of the long-range goals set by individuals in the front-line positions, an effective staffing system cannot meet its goals without the full understanding of the basic principles that the staffing system serves and its benefits for both the organization and the nursing department. An effective staffing system cannot survive without the full understanding, loyalty, and support of those individuals who will be implementing the system.

A staffing system must be compatible with the goals and philosophy of the nursing department in meeting its expectations for the quality of patient care and standards of nursing practice. In addition, for a staffing system to be functional and effective, it must meet the following five criteria:

1. A staffing system must enable the nursing administration to meet its goal hours per patient day.
2. A staffing system must be flexible.
3. A staffing system must provide a built-in justification system that can be utilized when the nursing hours per patient day do not meet the budget.
4. A staffing system must ensure some degree of effective utilization of nursing personnel.
5. A staffing system must leave a concise audit trail for nurse staffing patterns.

MEETING ESTABLISHED NURSING GOAL HOURS PER PATIENT DAY

It is hard to believe that, in an era when staffing systems capable of being computerized have become the state of the art in some institutions, a great number of nursing departments—nursing departments that pride themselves on providing the highest quality of patient care—still utilize the following equation:

$$\text{nursing goal hours per patient day} \times \text{number of patients} = \text{nursing hours required}$$

The hospital in Northern California for which this system was developed was no different. Before developing its current system, the staffing equation used was similar to the preceding equation. The result appeared more like the following:

$$\text{nursing goal hours per patient day} \times \text{number of patients} = \text{disaster}$$

This method for determining nurse staffing needs neglected to consider the patient's degree of illness or the competency and skill level of the nurse. The outcome of this pattern of staffing is illustrated in Exhibit 13-1. Patient care becomes fragmented; nursing personnel become disillusioned, quickly labeling their frustration as burnout rather than seeing the problem as one resolvable through adequate staffing allocations. A good staffing system will recognize that the job satisfaction of nursing personnel does not depend on nurse-to-patient ratios but rather on nurse-to-patient acuity ratios.

Exhibit 13-1 Results of Developing a Staffing System without Using a Patient Classification System

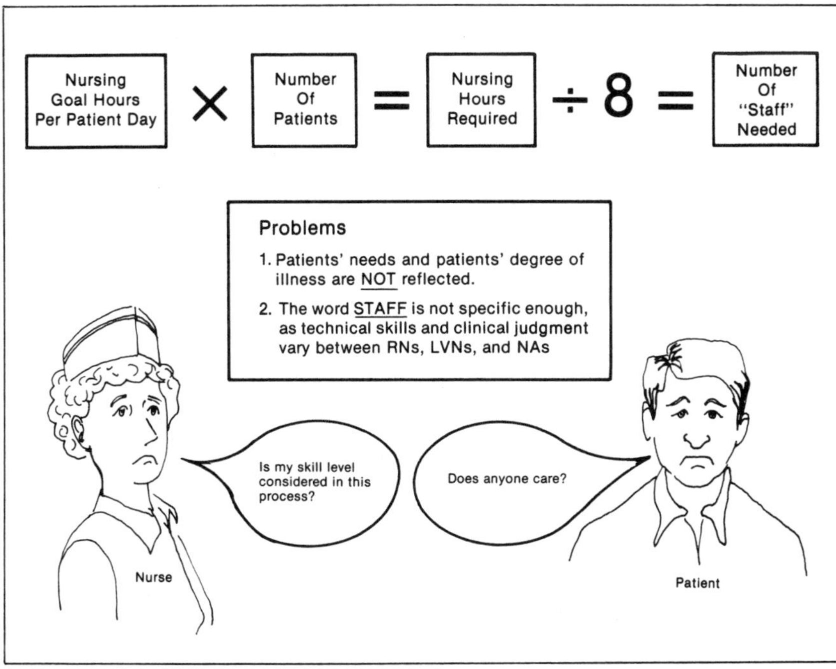

SYSTEM FLEXIBILITY AND A BUILT-IN JUSTIFICATION

As shown in Chapter 11, a patient classification system can be designed by assigning relative value units to each nursing activity. Nurse staffing policy is designed (Chapter 12) and each shift on each nursing unit can be staffed with position control (Chapter 14) as a baseline point. Any adjustments or reassignment of staff is based on the patient classification system and the total patient acuity as it applies to each nursing unit. The nursing administration determined through the time-and-motion studies described in Chapter 11 the maximum numbers of relative value units that a nurse can reasonably care for during each eight-hour shift. An example of this is shown in Table 13-1.

If the patient assignment range to each nurse exceeds the maximum relative value units allowed, this becomes the justifiable factor for redistributing nursing personnel from one unit to another. Likewise, if both units' average acuity exceeded the allowable maximum, this would serve as justification for calling in per-diem employees.

Table 13-1 Maximum Number of Relative Value Units

Shift	*Per Nurse*
Nights	115
Evenings	95
Days	75

An effective staffing system cannot be cast in concrete. Probably no other point needs to be emphasized more than the system's flexibility. Nursing managers are dealing with flexible and ever-changing entities: people, more specifically, nurses and patients. Probably no other profession contains a group of individuals who cry out louder for flexibility and autonomy.

Any staffing system must parallel the patient classification system. As the patient classification system fluctuates with acuity, so does the staffing system. For example, let's consider the situation in Table 13-2 for the day shift on two different med-surg nursing units, 1 South and 2 North.

The nursing administration has set its goals for nursing hours per patient day at 5.2 nursing hours per patient day (for one 24-hour period). The nursing administration has divided that 5.2 nursing hours per patient day so that each shift—days, evenings, and nights—has its own goal for nursing hours per patient shift. This has been further subdivided as in Table 13-3.

Table 13-2 Day-Shift Situation

Unit	*Patient Census*	*Total Patient Acuity*	*Average Patient Acuity*	*Number Staff Assigned*	*Average Acuity Assigned*
1 South	26	375	15	7	53.5
2 North	19	450	24	4	112.5

Table 13-3 Nursing Goals per Shift

Shift	*Nursing Hours Goal*
Nights	1.25
Days	2.20
Evenings	1.75
Total	5.20 nursing hours per patient day

Based on the information in Table 13-2 and the projected nursing goal hours in Table 13-3 one can calculate that the nursing hours for this day's shift will be 2.15 on 1 South nursing station and 1.68 on 2 North nursing station. To calculate this the number of staff assigned is multiplied by 8 hours worked in a shift, which equals the total hours worked. Then the total hours worked on the nursing station is divided by the patient census to arrive at the nursing hours for that shift:

$$\text{Number of staff} \times 8 \text{ hours worked} = \text{total hours worked}$$
$$\text{Total hours worked} \div \text{patient census} = \text{nursing hours per shift}$$

If the staffing is left as originally assigned, both nursing units would indeed meet their goal hours for the shift; in fact both units could enjoy a negative variance, that is, be operating below the goal for the unit. No doubt this would please the financial department of the hospital, but, as in Table 13-2, the acuity varies greatly between the two units, in fact, by 59 relative value units (112.5 − 53.5 = 59).

While the nursing staff on this day shift on 1 South will have average patient assignments consisting of 21.5 relative value units below the level of a maximum reasonable patient assignment (75 − 53.5 = 21.5), the nursing staff on 2 North will carry an average 37.5 relative value units over the reasonable level (112.5 − 75 = 37.5). The results can be inferior and fragmented patient care, with patient safety jeopardized. If the staffing were to remain as originally assigned, the nursing staff on 2 North would be overworked and probably irritated with the high acuity level of their patient assignments.

This situation becomes the basis for justification for the nursing supervisor to reassign or reallocate the nursing personnel. By reassigning two nurses from the 1 South unit to the 2 North unit, the average relative value unit assignment for each nurse would be 75 RVUs on both units, the goal of Table 13-1. While this solves the problem of uneven assignment of relative value units to the nursing staff, the nursing hours on this shift are altered so that 1 South will report 1.53 nursing hours for this shift (a negative variance) and 2 North will report 2.52 nursing hours for this shift (a positive variance). While 2 North will exceed its budgeted nursing hours, it is imperative that the nursing administration be able to make these adjustments in the staffing according to acuity and need and that the system allow for such flexibility. When the financial controller requests the justification for the elevated nursing hours on 2 North, the unit coordinator will be able to validate high patient acuity as the reason; the supervisor making the decision for reallocating the staff will be able to justify the rationale for redistributing staff from 1 South to 2 North.

In addition, the supervisor should document justification for *both* positive and negative variances. This documentation should occur consistently each time a variance in staffing is made. These documentation records should be kept on file in the nursing office and be readily available for the nursing administration to use not only for justifying the variances to the hospital controller but also for determining patterns where patient acuity may remain excessively high. The nursing administration may then be able to use a consistently high patient acuity on 2 North to justify the request for additional nursing hours per patient day in the next year's budget. Another important reason for keeping accurate records of staffing variances is to determine if a nursing unit is consistently reporting high patient acuity levels and potentially padding the system.

EFFECTIVE UTILIZATION OF NURSING PERSONNEL

A patient classification system and a staffing system, if properly modeled, should provide for the allocation of nursing personnel by matching the workload generated by patients' relative value units to a number of nursing personnel.[2] The selection of the category of personnel assigned to the nursing unit, that is, RNs, LVNs, and NAs, should vary from institution to institution, depending on the skill levels of each group as well as the individual performance capabilities. For example, in the facility where this system was designed the LVN category had been dramatically upgraded to include the skills of medication administration and a limited degree of IV therapy. In this same facility nearly all NA positions were upgraded with RNs or LVNs as NAs terminated employment, sought higher education, or transferred to other areas within the hospital. This simplified staffing in that there were more resources of professional nursing personnel and therefore a greater ability to blend staff more equally. Before a nursing department elects such a high percentage of professional staff personnel—in this case 72 percent RNs, 22 percent LVNs, 3 percent NAs, and 3 percent secretarial people (ward clerks)—nursing departments should study the cost effects of this process in addition to the availability of professional staff.

AN AUDIT TRAIL FOR FUTURE TRENDS

A nurse staffing system can provide nursing administration with a viable audit trail necessary to determine patient acuity, collect data, and project possible trends in nursing care relative to operational budgets. Through responsible monitoring of the staffing system, nursing managers can justify an overrun of a department's operational budget and can provide feedback data to support this justification to the hospital administrator and financial controller, thus demonstrating accountability.

In addition, if the hospital controller can develop a thorough understanding of the mechanics of the patient acuity system and staffing system, the controller would be able to measure the intensity factors relative to other departments. For example, if the lab or x-ray department were under its projected budgeted revenue

Exhibit 13-2 Using a Meaningful Patient Classification System to Meet and Justify Nursing Goal Hours

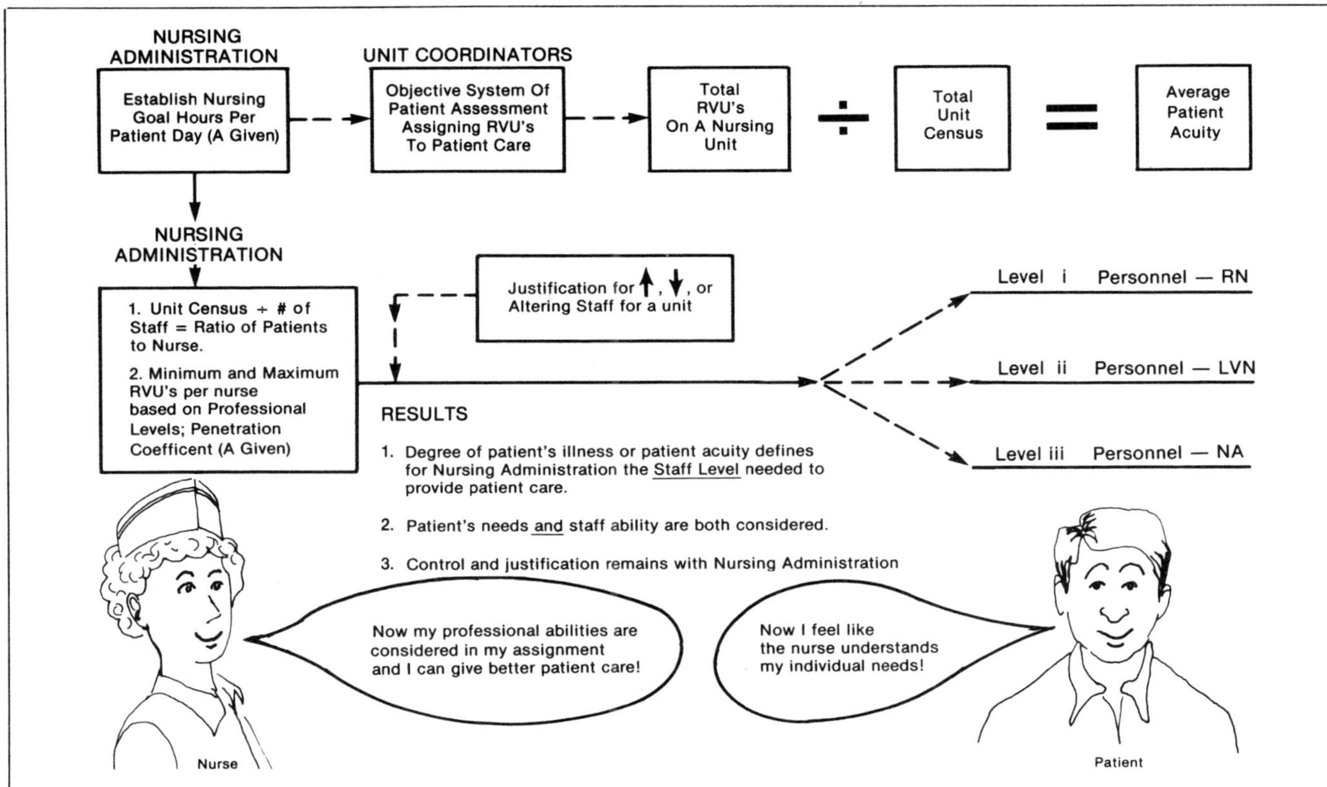

due to an under-budgeted number of procedures, the controller would be able to predict that the patient acuity on the nursing units is probably proportionately lower; concurrently high patient acuities generally indicate more critically ill patients who require more lab or x-ray procedures and tests. Likewise, if lab, x-ray, or even respiratory therapy experienced a high volume of procedures, one would expect to find an overall higher patient acuity throughout the nursing units.

A staffing system using patient acuities will not guarantee complete elimination of nurse staffing problems. But if a staffing system is soundly thought out, it can eliminate many of the traditional problems associated with nurse staffing. A good staffing system will better utilize the existing personnel and consider the needs of the patients and the skill level of the nurses, which certainly can have a positive effect on the nurses' job satisfaction. The staffing system should be flexible, have a built-in justification for both positive and negative variances in nursing hours, and act as a tool for the nursing department to reach its goal of nursing hours per patient day. Finally, a staffing system should include thorough documentation to:

- account for variances in staffing and
- show trends and patterns in patient acuities, which can be a valuable audit trail for projecting operating budgets.

While justification of additional nursing personnel is often a gray area that can be rationalized in many ways, nursing administrations need to emphasize the importance of utilizing consistent rational guides for adding staff. If the maximum number of acuity relative value units exceeds the recommended guidelines, as shown in Table 13-1, nurse dissatisfaction and patient complaints often increase as the direct result of the care that they did not receive, require, or expect.

The nursing department is not a revenue-producing department, other than generating a patient room charge. This can be a pitfall of staffing by an acuity system that is not based on the department's budget. In a system based on patient acuity the nursing department budget is based on nursing hours per patient day; this then becomes a mechanism to tie the acuity system into the budgeting process. In some larger facilities billing for nursing services provided is being formulated with some startling positive results. Goal hours can be met and staffing can successfully be accomplished through staffing mechanisms based on patient acuities. The results of staffing based on patient acuities show an increase in both patient and nurse satisfaction as described in Exhibit 13-2.

NOTES

1. Phyllis Giovanetti, "Understanding Patient Classification Systems," *Journal of Nursing Administration,* February 1979, p. 4.
2. Ibid.

Chapter 14

Executing the Patient Classification System through Position Control

OBJECTIVES

Following completion of this chapter the reader will be able to:

- define position control,
- calculate full-time equivalents,
- differentiate between productive time and nonproductive time as they relate to nursing hours,
- allocate staff according to classification and shift based on full-time equivalents, and
- determine vacant positions.

Why should one waste time developing a patient classification system if there isn't enough staff to care for the patients? This pessimistic question has been debated repeatedly. The financial administrator may enforce the nursing hours per patient day without totally accepting the nursing administration's justification for variations. If the nursing administration receives a deaf ear from the financial administration of the hospital, the mandated nursing hours per patient day elicit the same negative connotation from the nursing administration as acuity can from staff nurses. The only difference between the two groups is semantic; staff nurses want more bodies, while the nursing administration wants more hours. In both cases the requests equal more money in the eyes of financial administration. However, despite the most generous nursing hours per patient day, staffing shortages remain acute and staffing patterns inadequate. Perhaps the focal point of the problem is not necessarily one of nursing hours per patient day but rather one of position control.

Position control is the process by which the labor budget is developed and full-time equivalents (FTEs) are determined and maintained. One need not be a mathematical genius to calculate the labor budget. However, unless the process is followed step by step, grave repercussions could ensue (staffing shortages, inappropriate staff allocation, decreased staff morale, and poor patient care) regardless of the allotted nursing hours per patient day.

To understand position control better, let us select one unit and study the process step by step. At the completion of this exercise questions such as How many full-time equivalents do I need? How do I account for nonproductive time? How many staff members do I need every day, every shift? will have been answered.

DETERMINING FTEs

One South is a 34-bed unit. Both preoperative and postoperative patients are admitted to this particular unit. The facility is far too small to specialize according to diagnosis and surgical procedure. Consequently, the staff on 1 South caters to a wide variety of surgical patients (orthopedic, thoracic, vascular, etc.). As Janet, the unit coordinator, starts to prepare her budget she must determine if the type of services rendered, the practice of nursing modalities, or the profile of patients on her unit will change over the next year. Perhaps open heart surgery will be offered at this facility or the practice of primary nursing will be introduced. Factors such as these must be considered in developing the budget for the next fiscal year. In this case neither the nursing administration nor Janet have made any plans to introduce any drastic change on 1 South. Janet begins the budgeting process by projecting the estimated occupancy rate for the next year based on last year's actual patient days.

To determine the estimated occupancy rate, Janet will review last year's monthly census reports. These reports reflect the actual census according to each 28-day accounting period. Also visible in this monthly report are patterns of high and low census periods.

JAN.	1	2	3	4	5	6	7	8	9	10	11	12	13	DEC.
	770	760	750	790	780	770	750	745	750	770	760	765	760	

The total patient days (9,920) is divided by the number of accounting periods (13), yielding the average patient days per accounting period (763.08). By dividing the average patient days per accounting period (763.08) by the number of days in an accounting period (28), Janet is able to determine the average patient days or average unit of service per day (27.25). Janet then reviews the growth that 1 South has experienced historically (3 percent). She and the financial administrator project a 5 percent increase in daily patient days for the upcoming year. Janet multiplies the current average patient days (27.25) by the growth factor (5 percent) to determine the estimated projected increase in patients per day (1.36). The sum of the current average patient days (27.25) and the projected increase in patient days (1.36) equals the average daily patient days/units of service (28.61) projected for the next fiscal year. By dividing the average daily patient days (28.61) by the total number of beds available on 1 South (34), Janet is able to confirm an estimated occupancy rate of 84 percent.

Now that Janet has calculated the average patient days, she obtains the nursing care hours per patient day from the nursing administration, which in the case of 1 South is 5.2 nursing care hours per patient day. The nursing care hours per patient day represents the number of hours required by each nurse, each day, to perform the nursing activities necessary to care for any given patient adequately. In other words a nursing unit budgeted at 5.5 nursing hours per patient day expects that 5.5 hours of direct nursing time per 24 hours will be expended caring for one patient. Hours per patient day is based on historical data obtained from time-and-motion studies, current trends of hospitals with similar size and services offered, and local competition.

Janet's next step is to determine the number of hours required as well as the number of staff required to care for the projected number of patients on a daily basis. To arrive at the daily hours required (148.77), Janet multiplies the average patient days (28.61) by the hours per patient day (5.2). Next the daily hours required (148.77) is divided by the number of hours in one shift (8) to determine the number of staff required daily to care for the patients (18.60).

PRODUCTIVE VERSUS NONPRODUCTIVE TIME

Janet begins to wonder about productive versus nonproductive time (Table 14-1). As Janet says, "With the hours per patient day as they are, I hardly have enough staff to cover productive time let alone nonproductive time." She directs her attention to nonproductive time: weekend days off, educational leave, holidays, vacation, and sick leave. The nursing staff on her unit alternate working weekends. Hence, there are 104 weekend days off per employee. Holiday leave equals 9 days while educational leave equals 5 days. The average vacation time and sick time equal 15 days and 5 days, respectively. The sum of all nonproductive time is 138 days.

Therefore, by subtracting the nonproductive time (138) from the total number of work days in a year (365), the actual number of work days (or productive time) is determined (227). Janet calculates her FTE ratio (1.61) by dividing the number of work days in a year (365) by the number of actual work days (227). This full-time equivalent ratio represents the number of FTEs required to cover both productive and nonproductive time for one full-time employee.

Table 14-1 Nonproductive Time

104	Weekend days off
9	Holidays
5	Educational leave
15	Vacation days
5	Sick days
138	Nonproductive time
365	Total work
−138	Nonproductive time
227	Productive time

365 work days in a year ÷ 227 (productive time) = 1.61 (FTE ratio)

ASSIGNING SHIFTS

Janet puts these figures aside and unplugs her calculator for a while. She begins to develop a daily staffing plan based on an average daily census of 28.61, knowing that 18.60 staff members have been allotted to her unit on a daily basis. Janet must decide how many staff members are to be allocated to each respective shift. Just as the hours per patient days is influenced by historical data and current trends, so too is the number of staff members per shift. Realistically Janet cannot simply allocate 50 percent of the staff to the day shift, 30 percent of the staff to the evening shift, and the remaining 20 percent to the night shift because these percentages (or any other, for that matter) sound reasonable. Arbitrary allocation of staff may only compound the problems for the nursing administrator and the nursing staff.

Gross imbalances of staff allocation per shift will only pit one shift against the other. Instead of the staff working together as a cohesive group 24 hours a day, the group tends to work as three separate teams 8 hours a day. Continuity of care becomes fragmented, the quality of care is jeopardized, and the morale of the staff takes a nose dive. Again complaints begin to surface from the physicians, the nurses, and the patients. Again the nursing administration encounters dissatisfaction from the workers and the consumers. Granted, trial and error is involved in allocation of staff per shift. However, a certain percentage can be determined whereby the continuity of care, the quality of care, and the staff morale are not jeopardized.

Janet finds herself considering other factors influencing staff allocation by shift. For instance, many of the medical staff meetings (department of medicine and department of surgery) are conducted on the hospital premises in the early evening. Inevitably physicians make rounds either before or after their meetings. In addition, the offices of many of the physicians are located across the street. Their close proximity and easy accessibility to the hospital make early evening rounds a reality. Consequently the evening shift may experience as much physician traffic as the day shift.

Medication times will also influence staff allocation. For example, facility A may designate Q 6 hour times as 6-12-6-12, facility B may designate the times as 5-11-5-11, and facility C may designate the times as 9-3-9-3. The designated shift times of each facility will further influence the staff allocation. Shift times at facility A are 7:30 A.M.–4 P.M., 3:30 P.M.–midnight, and 11:30 P.M.–8 A.M.; shift times at facility B are 7 A.M.–3:30 P.M., 3 P.M.–11:30 P.M., and 11 P.M.–7:30 A.M.; and shift times at facility C are 7:30 A.M.–4 P.M., 3:30 P.M.–midnight, and 11:30 P.M.–8 A.M. When the medication times are then correlated with the shift times of the three facilities, it becomes evident that the number of medications to be administered can affect one shift more than the other as Table 14-2 indicates.

If at facility A the patient is to receive two grams of Keflin every 6 hours, the night shift is responsible for administering two doses of the medication (midnight and 6 A.M.) while both the day and evening shifts are responsible for administering only one dose of the medication. In contrast both doses at facility B will be administered by the evening shift, while at facility C both doses of the medication will be administered by the day shift. In all these cases, the staff allocation should be in conjunction with the times when medications are to be administered.

After considering these factors, it became apparent to Janet that the staff allocation per shift was unreasonable and unrealistic. Janet began to juggle the percentages. Eventually, after weeks of trial and error, she was able to establish a more reasonable and realistic staffing plan. Her daily staffing plan is plotted in Table 14-3.

Table 14-2 Medication and Shift Times

	Facility A				*Facility B*				*Facility C*		
	7:30A 4:00P	*3:30P 12:00M*	*11:30P 8:00A*		*7:00A 3:30P*	*3:00P 11:30P*	*11:00P 7:30A*		*7:30A 4:00P*	*3:30P 12:00M*	*11:30P 8:00A*
6AM			1	5AM			1	3AM			1
12N	1			11AM	1			9AM	1		
6PM		1		5PM		1		3PM	1		
12MN			1	11PM		1		9PM		1	

Table 14-3 Daily Staffing Plan

Staff	Day	Evening	Night	Total
Unit coordinator	1	0	0	1.00
Charge nurse	0	1	1	2.00
Staff nurse	3	3	2.0	8.00
LVN/LPN	3	2	1.6	6.60
Nurse's aide	0	0	0	0.00
Ward clerk/secretary	1	0	0	1.00
Daily shift total	8	6	4.6	18.60

Since 18.60 staff members represents 5.2 hours per patient day, it is necessary to determine the hours per patient day allotted to each shift (Table 14-4). To determine the hours per patient day per shift, Janet must first divide the daily shift totals by 18.60. Dividing 8, 6, and 4.6 by 18.60 yields 43, 32, and 25. These figures are actual percentages allotted to each shift. In other words 43 percent of the staff is allotted to the day shift, 32 percent to the evening shift, and 25 percent to the night shift. To convert these percentages into hours per patient day per shift, Janet must multiply 5.2 by 43 percent, 32 percent, and 25 percent. The figures obtained (2.2, 1.7, and 1.3) represent the hours per patient day for the day, evening, and night shifts, respectively.

Like the 5.2 hours per patient day, these figures also indicate the amount of nursing time expended on one patient on each respective shift. By juggling the percentages and readjusting the hours per patient day per shift, Janet was able to avoid fragmented patient care, thereby improving the quality of care rendered. Complaints from physicians, nurses, and patients decreased. Friction among staff members and between shifts also decreased. This is not to imply that perfection has been attained; rather the nursing administration and Janet heard the complaints, registered the complaints, addressed the friction, and sought a better

Table 14-4 Hours per Patient Day per Shift

Shift	Percentage per Shift	Hours per Shift
Day	$\frac{8}{18.60} = 43\%$	$43\% \times 5.2 = 2.2$
Evening	$\frac{6}{18.60} = 32\%$	$32\% \times 5.2 = 1.7$
Night	$\frac{4.6}{18.60} = 25\%$	$25\% \times 5.2 = 1.3$

18.6 staff members = 5.2 hours per patient day

solution. Furthermore, these percentages are not the ultimate, for they will need to be changed and altered.

Janet's next step is to determine patient-staff ratios. On 1 South the unit coordinator and the evening charge nurse do not deliver bedside nursing care; the night charge nurse functions as both charge nurse and staff nurse. The unit clerk (secretary) is responsible for ordering supplies, transcribing doctors' orders, answering telephones, etc. The clerk does not deliver bedside nursing care. In other words the number of people actually delivering bedside nursing care on days, evenings, and nights are 6, 5, and 4.6, respectively. Dividing the average daily patient days (28.61) by the number of staff delivering bedside nursing care will yield the patient/staff ratio (Table 14-5).

FTE STAFF BY CLASSIFICATION

It's time to return to the aid of the calculator again. Janet needs to determine the FTE staff according to classification (Table 14-6). First and foremost, she must determine the combined productive and nonproductive FTE (29.94) by multiplying the daily staff required (18.60) by the FTE ratio (1.61). Second, she must differentiate between basic FTE and vacation, holiday and sick (VHS) FTE, also known as nonproductive FTE. To ascertain the portion of the FTE ratio that pertains to productive time, first she subtracts the weekend days (104) from the total days in the year (365). The figure obtained (261) is then divided into the total days in the year (365). This calculation (1.4), therefore, yields the basic coverage needed to operate the facility 7 days a week and 24 hours a day.

The basic coverage, or productive FTE ratio, can be explained in another way. An individual hired as a full-time employee (1.0) works 80 hours in a 14-day period. These 80 hours constitute 10 working days. Therefore, to cover the remaining days in the 14-day period, Janet needs an employee to work 4 days. This employee (0.4) combined with the full-time employee (1.0) equals the basic productive FTE ratio of 1.4. To determine the nonproductive FTE ratio needed to cover vacation, holiday, sick, and educational days (0.21), one merely subtracts 1.4 from 1.61. Multiplying the daily staff required (18.60) by 1.40 and by 0.21 yields the total basic FTE (26.04) and the total VHS FTE (3.90), respectively.

Table 14-5 Patient/Staff Ratios

	Days	*Evenings*	*Nights*
Number of staff	6	5	4.6
Number of patients	28.61	28.61	28.61
Patient/staff ratios	4/4/5/5/5/5	5/5/6/6/6	7/7/7/7/

In order to convert staff according to classification into FTEs, further calculation is necessary. Essentially, by multiplying the total number of staff according to classification by both the basic FTE (1.40) and the VHS FTE (0.21), one can arrive at the total FTE by classification. For example, Janet has requested 8 RNs to staff her unit on a 24-hour basis. Multiplying the total RNs needed (8) by the basic FTE (1.40) yields the FTE required (11.20) to cover the basic 7-day work week while multiplying the total RNs needed (8) by the VHS FTE (0.21) yields the FTE required (1.68) to cover nonproductive time. Table 14-7 indicates the informational results achieved in this process.

Table 14-6 Determination of FTE Staff

18.60	Daily staff required
× 1.61	FTE ratio
29.94	Total productive & nonproductive FTE

365	Total work days in a year
− 104	Weekend days off
261	Productive days

365 ÷ 261 Productive days = 1.4 (basic FTE)

1.61	FTE ratio
− 1.40	Basic productive FTE
0.21	Nonproductive/vacation, holiday, sick FTE

18.60	Daily staff	18.60	Daily staff
× 1.40	Basic FTE	× 0.21	VHS FTE
26.04	Total basic FTE	3.90	Total VHS FTE

Table 14-7 Staff by Classification

Staff Member	*Staff by Classification*				*FTE Staff by Classification*		
	Days	*Eves*	*NOCS*	*Total*	*Basic*	*VHS*	*Total*
Unit coordinator	1	0	0	1	1.40	0.21	1.61
Charge nurse	0	1	1	2	2.80	0.42	3.22
Staff nurse	3	3	2	8	11.20	1.68	12.88
LVN/LPN	3	2	1.6	6.6	9.24	1.38	10.62
Nurse's aide	0	0	0	0	0	0	0
Ward clerk	1	0	0	1	1.40	0.21	1.61
Daily total staff	8	6	4.6	18.6	26.04	3.90	29.94

It is not enough simply to differentiate between the basic and VHS FTE only according to classification. A similar process must be followed in order to allocate staff according to each shift. Once again Janet has requested that 6 staff members cover the evening shift on a daily basis. As a result of multiplying the number of staff members requested (6) by the basic FTE (1.40) and the VHS FTE (0.21), Janet is able to differentiate between productive time (8.4) and nonproductive time (1.26) on the evening shift. Thus, the total FTE required to staff the evening shift is 9.66. Completion of this process yielded the results in Table 14-8.

FINAL STAFFING PLAN

At last, Janet is approaching the final step in identifying position control needs. That step is neither easier nor less tedious than any of the previous steps. Janet refers to her daily staffing plan. On the day shift she would like 4 RNs (1 unit coordinator and 3 staff nurses), 3 LVNs, and 1 ward clerk on duty every day. She calculates productive and nonproductive time according to classification. For instance, 4 RNs multiplied by the basic FTE (1.40) and the VHS FTE (0.21) yields 5.60 FTE and 0.84 FTE, respectively. Thus, in order to staff the day shift Janet needs 6.44 FTE at the RN level. The figures in Table 14-9 represent Janet's calculations of FTEs needed per shift and per classification.

Table 14-8 FTE Staff by Shift

FTE Personnel	*Days*	*Eves*	*NOCS*	*Total*
Basic 7-day week coverage	11.20	8.40	6.44	26.04
Vac. hol. sick coverage	1.68	1.26	0.96	3.90
Total FTE personnel	12.88	9.66	7.40	29.94

Table 14-9 FTEs per Shift and Classification

	Days			*Evenings*			*Nights*		
	RN	*LVN*	*WC*	*RN*	*LVN*	*WC*	*RN*	*LVN*	*WC*
Basic FTE	5.60	4.20	1.40	5.60	2.80	--	4.20	2.24	--
VHS FTE	0.84	0.63	0.21	0.84	0.42	--	0.63	0.33	--
Total FTE	6.44	4.83	1.61	6.44	3.22	--	4.83	2.57	--

These figures are transcribed to the position control form (Exhibit 14-1). Janet must decide how many full-time versus part-time positions are warranted. The rule of thumb that has worked well for Janet is quite simple: every full-time position should be complemented by a part-time position. Furthermore Janet must keep in mind weekend coverage because only half of the staff is available for weekend duty. She must divide the FTEs to coincide with the master daily staffing plan. Janet chooses to distribute the FTEs as illustrated in Exhibit 14-1.

Exhibit 14-1 Position Control Form

UC 1.0 Janet	RN 1.0 Mary	RN 1.0 Terry	RN 1.0 Cheryl	RN 0.6 Kathy	RN 0.6 Eileen
RN 0.6 Maureen	RN 0.6 Karen			LVN 1.0 Pat	LVN 1.0 Carol
LVN 1.0 Mary	LVN 0.6 Phyllis	LVN 0.6 Jeanette	LVN 0.6 Linda		WC 1.0 Sheila

CN 1.0 Marilyn	RN 1.0 Marina	RN 1.0 Jill	RN 1.0 Laurel	RN 0.6 Ellen	RN 0.6 Renee
RN 0.6 Esther	RN 0.6 Diane				
LVN 1.0 Linda	LVN 1.0 Evelyn	LVN 0.6 Paula	LVN 0.6		

CN 1.0 Elizabeth	RN 0.8 Ann	RN 0.8 Elaine	RN 0.8 Peggy	RN 0.8	RN 0.6 Pamela
LVN 1.0 Kathy	LVN 0.8 Susan	LVN 0.8			

	DAYS			EVENINGS			NIGHTS		
	RN	LVN	WC	RN	LVN	WC	RN	LVN	WC
BASIC FTE	5.60	4.20	1.40	5.60	2.80	-	4.20	2.24	-
VHS FTE	.84	.63	.21	.84	.42	-	.63	.33	-
TOTAL FTE	6.44	4.83	1.61	6.44	3.22	-	4.83	2.57	-
REAL FTE	6.40	4.80	1.00	6.40	3.20	-	4.00	1.80	-
VARIANCE	.04	.03	.61	.04	.02	-	.83	.77	-

Source: Reprinted with permission of Nursing Department, Doctors Hospital of Pinole, Pinole, California.

Although the FTEs are not evenly distributed according to both the daily staffing plan and the stated rule of thumb, Janet does provide reasonable justification for these variations. As unit coordinator, Janet is not obligated to work on the weekends. As a result, there is an uneven division of RNs available for weekend duty—with four on one weekend and three on the opposite weekend. Cognizant of this, Janet opts to maintain this particular staffing plan because historically the census on 1 South is reduced significantly every Friday and Saturday, thereby decreasing the staffing needs proportionally. On the night shift Janet's staffing pattern does not quite complement every full-time position with a part-time position. In fact, it appears as if there is an overabundance of part-time personnel. Janet considers two major points contributing to this situation. First, she recognizes that recruitment of personnel for *any* night shift position is a difficult task in her facility. Second, she recognizes that the goal for recruitment of full-time personnel for that particular shift is equally difficult. Janet considers both points and distributes the FTEs accordingly. Finally, Janet enters the names and statuses of the current personnel into the appropriate boxes and is able to identify her staffing needs readily. Janet has completed position control for 1 South based on 5.2 nursing hours per patient day for a projected daily census of 28.61.

Why did Janet calculate her position control only on the projected average daily census? Surely there will be days when the census falls above or below the projection. For instance, how many FTEs are required for a census of 20, 24, or 32? How does the daily staffing plan for a census of 20, 24, or 32 differ from the staffing plan based on a census of 28.61?

In reality, Janet does not calculate position control based only on the projected average daily census. Janet uses the projected average daily census as a focal point on which to base her staffing plan and her subsequent scheduling pattern. It is this focal point for which Janet must budget and maintain adequate FTEs. It is hardly worthwhile to budget for a census of 34 when such a census cannot be maintained. The end result is far too many FTEs, exorbitant costs, and uncontrollable layoffs. Conversely, to budget for any census below 28.61 is not without its drawbacks. Rather than too many FTEs, Janet will experience an acute shortage of FTEs. Consequently costs will escalate as the budgeted, available staff members work overtime and double shifts. Per-diem and registry utilization will also increase; this will escalate costs even more. Finally, the nursing staff will experience fatigue, frustration, and burnout.

This is not to say that Janet should ignore any census above or below 28.61. Quite the contrary, Janet should develop position control for each individual census whether it falls above or below the projected average daily census. The important point is that FTEs should be based on the projected average daily census and personnel hired accordingly. Not only is Janet responsible for maintaining appropriate FTEs; she is also responsible for flexing the FTEs to correspond with any deviations from the projection. The only way in which this can be done is by

Janet knowing the exact number of staff warranted for the varying censuses. Table 14-10 indicates the results of position control for every census. Furthermore, it also indicates the 43 percent, 32 percent, and 25 percent allocation of staff per shift. In this way the hours per patient day and hours per patient day per shift remain constant.

Although the results of position control presented in Table 14-10 address only numbers, one major point needs to be emphasized. Janet has discovered that for a census above 28 she may actually operate below the budgeted hours per patient day. Both she and the staff have noted that the average patient acuity is lowest during high census days. This is not to suggest the absence of high-acuity patients; rather it appears that during high census days a number of low-acuity patients seem to offset the impact of high-acuity patients. Hence, during high census periods Janet is generally able to operate well below her budget.

The authors strongly encourage this endeavor because the opposite situation may present itself during low census days. Historical data retrieved from the daily

Table 14-10 Census-Based Position Control

HPPD	CENSUS	STAFF	DAYS = 43%/2.2	PMS = 32%/1.7	NOCS = 25%/1.3
5.2	34	22.10	9.50	7.07	5.53
5.2	33	21.45	9.22	6.86	5.36
5.2	32	20.80	8.94	6.66	5.20
5.2	31	20.15	8.66	6.45	5.04
5.2	30	19.50	8.39	6.24	4.88
5.2	29	18.85	8.11	6.03	4.71
5.2	28	18.20	7.83	5.82	4.55
5.2	27	17.55	7.55	5.62	4.39
5.2	26	16.90	7.27	5.41	4.23
5.2	25	16.25	6.99	5.20	4.06
5.2	24	15.60	6.71	4.99	3.90
5.2	23	14.95	6.43	4.78	3.74
5.2	22	14.30	6.15	4.58	3.58
5.2	21	13.65	5.87	4.37	3.41
5.2	20	13.00	5.59	4.16	3.25
5.2	19	12.35	5.31	3.95	3.09
5.2	18	11.70	5.03	3.74	2.93
5.2	17	11.05	4.75	3.54	2.76
5.2	16	10.40	4.47	3.33	2.60
5.2	15	9.75	4.19	3.12	2.44
5.2	14	9.10	3.91	2.91	2.28
5.2	13	8.45	3.63	2.70	2.11
5.2	12	7.80	3.35	2.50	1.95
5.2	11	7.15	3.07	2.29	1.79
5.2	10	6.50	2.80	2.08	1.63
5.2	9	5.85	2.52	1.87	1.46
5.2	8	5.20	2.24	1.66	1.30
5.2	7	4.55	1.96	1.46	1.14
5.2	6	3.90	1.68	1.25	0.98
5.2	5	3.25	1.40	1.04	0.81
5.2	4	2.60	1.12	0.83	0.65
5.2	3	1.95	0.84	0.62	0.49
5.2	2	1.30	0.56	0.42	0.33
5.2	1	0.65	0.28	0.21	0.16

nursing office reports suggest that as the census decreases, the average patient acuity increases. To some extent then, patient census and patient acuity are inversely related. For a census of 9 with an average patient acuity of 20, Janet cannot possibly deliver patient care with 2.5 staff members. Under these circumstances, Janet will need at least 1 additional staff member. By operating below the budget during high census periods when possible, Janet is able to counterbalance the budget when she must operate above the budget during low-census, above-average acuity periods. "Massaging" the budget in this manner will justify and allow Janet the flexibility to staff according to patient care needs. Perhaps for the month of February Janet will be over budget due to the low-census, high-acuity days. However, her year-to-date expenses and costs run a greater chance of coinciding with the actual budget as a result of reducing staff during high-census, low- to average-acuity periods. In this way a more realistic and reasonable staffing pattern can be achieved while simultaneously preventing direct insult to the budget.

In conclusion, the authors encourage developing and formulating an individual position control system. This process is a tedious task but necessary. Nursing managers recognize that they cannot bury heads in the sand any longer. Just as the staff nurses must deal with relative value units, so too must nursing administrators and nursing middle managers accept and deal with nursing hours per patient day, FTEs, and budgetary projections.

Daily staffing patterns, patient/staff ratios, and RN/LVN ratios ought to be determined by the nursing administration with only figurative and mathematical consultative input from financial administration, hospital administration, or even a corporate administration. While these groups can offer advice and figurative expertise, the nursing administration must insist that the input remain advice, and not mandates. Nursing administrations must learn to deal with the numbers, speak the language of the financial administrator, and seek advice or input when appropriate, while maintaining the control and accepting the responsibility for the outcome of the staffing system and position control.

Even with adequate nursing hours per patient day allotted, acute staffing shortages can result if position control is not developed. Without position control there is no method to determine how FTEs are to be distributed among all three shifts for the seven days in a week. A good position control system can ultimately pave the way for appropriate staff allocation. Exhibits 14-2 and 14-3 can aid in the development of personal position control.

Exhibit 14-2 Position Control Equations

1. $$\frac{\text{TOTAL PATIENT DAYS}}{\text{NUMBER OF ACCOUNTING PERIODS}} = \text{AVERAGE PATIENT DAYS PER ACCOUNTING PERIOD}$$

2. $$\frac{\text{AVERAGE PATIENT DAYS PER ACCOUNTING PERIOD}}{\text{NUMBER OF DAYS PER ACCOUNTING PERIOD}} = \text{AVERAGE PATIENT DAYS OR UNIT OF SERVICE}$$

3. AVERAGE PATIENT DAYS PER DAY × GROWTH FACTOR = PROJECTED INCREASE IN PATIENTS PER DAY

4. AVERAGE PATIENT DAYS + PROJECTED INCREASE IN PATIENTS PER DAY = AVERAGE DAILY PATIENT DAYS FOR THE FISCAL YEAR

5. $$\frac{\text{AVERAGE DAILY PATIENT DAYS}}{\text{TOTAL NUMBER OF BEDS ON THE UNIT}} = \text{ESTIMATED OCCUPANCY RATE}$$

6. AVERAGE PATIENT DAYS × HOURS PER PATIENT DAY = DAILY HOURS REQUIRED

7. $$\frac{\text{DAILY HOURS REQUIRED}}{\text{NUMBER OF HOURS PER SHIFT}} = \text{DAILY STAFF REQUIRED}$$

8. NUMBER OF WORK DAYS PER YEAR − NUMBER OF NONPRODUCTIVE DAYS PER YEAR = NUMBER OF ACTUAL WORK DAYS

9. $$\frac{\text{NUMBER OF WORK DAYS PER YEAR}}{\text{NUMBER OF ACTUAL WORK DAYS}} = \text{FULL TIME EQUIVALENT RATIO}$$

10. DAILY STAFF REQUIRED × FTE RATIO = TOTAL FTE

11. $\dfrac{\text{TOTAL DAYS IN A YEAR}}{\text{TOTAL DAYS IN A YEAR} - \text{WEEKEND DAYS}}$ = PRODUCTIVE OR BASIC FTE

12. TOTAL FTE − PRODUCTIVE OR BASIC FTE = VHS FTE

13. $\dfrac{\text{TOTAL FTE}}{\text{DAILY STAFF REQUIRED}}$ = FTE PER EMPLOYEE

14. FTE PER EMPLOYEE − PRODUCTIVE OR BASIC FTE PER EMPLOYEE = VHS FTE PER EMPLOYEE

15. TOTAL NUMBER OF STAFF PER CLASSIFICATION × PRODUCTIVE OR BASIC FTE = PRODUCTIVE OR BASIC FTE STAFF PER CLASSIFICATION

16. TOTAL NUMBER OF STAFF PER CLASSIFICATION × VHS FTE = VHS FTE STAFF PER CLASSIFICATION

17. TOTAL NUMBER OF STAFF PER SHIFT × PRODUCTIVE OR BASIC FTE = PRODUCTIVE OR BASIC FTE STAFF PER SHIFT

18. TOTAL NUMBER OF STAFF PER SHIFT × VHS FTE = VHS FTE STAFF PER SHIFT

19. TOTAL NUMBER OF STAFF PER CLASSIFICATION PER SHIFT × PRODUCTIVE FTE = PRODUCTIVE FTE STAFF PER CLASSIFICATION PER SHIFT

20. TOTAL NUMBER OF STAFF PER CLASSIFICATION PER SHIFT × VHS FTE = VHS FTE STAFF PER CLASSIFICATION PER SHIFT

Source: Reprinted with permission of Nursing Department, Doctors Hospital of Pinole, Pinole, California.

Exhibit 14-3 Full-Time Equivalent Form

UNIT ________ FISCAL YEAR ________ PREPARED BY: ________________ APPROVED BY: ________________

UNIT OF SERVICE ________________ BEDS AVAILABLE _______ OCCUPANCY RATE _______ HOURS PER DAY ____

AVERAGE DAILY UNITS OF SERVICE ____ DAILY HOURS REQUIRED ____ DAILY STAFF REQUIRED ____

WEEKEND DAYS OFF ____ VACATION ____ HOLIDAY ____ SICK LEAVE ____ EDUCATIONAL LEAVE _____

TOTAL DAYS NOT WORKED ____
ACTUAL WORK DAYS ____

FTE RATIO ____ FTE TOTAL ____ BASIC FTE ____ VHS FTE ____

DAILY STAFFING PLAN					FTE STAFF BY CLASSIFICATION		
CLASSIFICATION	DAYS	EVENINGS	NIGHTS	TOTALS	BASIC	VHS	TOTAL
UNIT COORDINATOR							
CHARGE NURSE							
STAFF NURSE							
LVN/LPN							
NURSES AIDE							
WARD CLERK							
TOTAL DAILY STAFF							

FTE PERSONNEL:	DAYS	EVENINGS	NIGHTS	TOTAL
BASIC COVERAGE:				
VHS COVERAGE				
TOTAL FTE COVERAGE				

Source: Reprinted with permission of Nursing Department, Doctors Hospital of Pinole, Pinole, California.

Chapter 15

Scheduling—An Integral Part of Position Control

OBJECTIVES

Following completion of this chapter the reader will be able to:

- correlate scheduling with the daily master staffing plan,
- examine the role of the per-diem/short-hour nurse in relationship to the daily staffing plan, and
- identify alternative scheduling methods that may enhance the daily staffing plan.

The development of position control is dependent on the science of mathematics. A byproduct of position control, scheduling, also remains dependent on the science of basic mathematical principles. Scheduling is not, and should not be, an entity in and of itself. Rather, it must be directly correlated with the daily staffing plan developed through position control. If the process of scheduling remains separated from position control, all Janet's efforts toward coordinating a semblance of position control (Chapter 14) have been in vain.

Many factors affect scheduling, such as vacations, illnesses, educational leaves, and fluctuating patient census. However, all these factors were taken into consideration when Janet developed position control based on the unit's specific projected average daily census. Subsequently Janet's schedule must be reflective of her daily staffing plan based on that same average daily census. Janet realizes that scheduling is not an easy task. If anything, it is both an art and a science that requires intricate workmanship within the confines of established boundaries (position control).

A WORKABLE SCHEDULE

To develop a workable schedule, Janet refers to the daily staffing plan, which was based on a projected average daily census of 28.61 patients. Division of the daily staffing plan is shown in Table 15-1.

For simplicity and time, let us focus on a two-week schedule patterned for the day shift staff. Janet would ultimately like to schedule four RNs, three LVNs, and one ward clerk on a daily basis. Her initial step is to plot her schedule according to the desired level and status, as illustrated in Exhibit 15-1.

Since all unit coordinators generally work Monday through Friday while other employees in Janet's unit are granted every other weekend off, Janet's next step is to schedule her staff according to weekend commitments. Obviously the weekend of the 7th and 8th fall short of Janet's daily staffing needs as only three RNs are available for work as compared to the weekend when four RNs are scheduled. To supplement her daily staffing plan, Janet considers several options.

Janet might decide to work every other weekend. Some staff members would support such an endeavor. Janet has volunteered her services when patient census and patient acuity remained exceptionally high. Although Janet enjoys her weekends off, she has justifiable reasons for not scheduling herself every other weekend on a permanent basis. As unit coordinator Janet is responsible for the overall planning, organizing, directing, controlling, and evaluating of the nursing care and the personnel on her unit. Her activities include, but are not limited to, supervising direct patient care; promoting and participating in staff, patient, and family education; executing and delegating physicians' orders; rendering direct patient care in selected situations; controlling inventory and supplies; preparing both the capital and operating budgets; completing written performance evaluations on all staff members; and attending meetings as directed by the nursing administrator. Such broad responsibilities and activities are dependent on consistency and stamina. To expect Janet to fulfill the objectives of her job description while submitting herself to a fluctuating schedule would be highly impractical.

Table 15-1 Daily Staffing Plan

Staff	*Day*	*Evening*	*Night*	*24-Hour Total*
Unit coordinator	1	0	0	1
Charge nurse	0	1	1	2
Staff nurse (RN)	3	3	2	8
LVN/LPN	3	2	1.6	6.6
Nurse's aide	-	-	-	-
Ward clerk	1	0	0	1
Daily staff total	8	6	4.6	18.6

Exhibit 15-1 Nursing Department Schedule—1 South

REGISTERED NURSES		SUN 1	MON 2	TUE 3	WED 4	THU 5	FRI 6	SAT 7	SUN 8	MON 9	TUE 10	WED 11	THU 12	FRI 13	SAT 14
JANET	1.0	X						X	X						X
MARY	1.0	X			X					X					X
TERRY	1.0				X			X	X					X	
CHERYL	1.0			X				X	X				X		
KATHY	0.6	X	X			X	X			X	X	X			X
EILEEN	0.6	X	X			X	X			X	X	X			X
MAUREEN	0.6		X	X			X	X	X			X	X	X	
KAREN	0.6		X	X			X	X	X			X	X	X	

LIC. VOC. NURSES		SUN 1	MON 2	TUE 3	WED 4	THU 5	FRI 6	SAT 7	SUN 8	MON 9	TUE 10	WED 11	THU 12	FRI 13	SAT 14
PAT	1.0	X				X				X					X
CAROL	1.0	X					X				X				X
DONNA	1.0			X				X	X				X		
PHYLLIS	0.6		X	X			X	X	X			X	X	X	
JOAN	0.6		X	X	X			X	X	X			X	X	
LINDA	0.6	X			X	X	X			X	X	X			X

WARD CLERK		SUN 1	MON 2	TUE 3	WED 4	THU 5	FRI 6	SAT 7	SUN 8	MON 9	TUE 10	WED 11	THU 12	FRI 13	SAT 14
SHEILA	1.0	X				X					X				X
TOTALS	RN/LVN/WC	4/3/0	4/4/1	5/3/1	6/4/1	6/4/0	4/3/1	3/3/1	3/3/1	5/3/1	6/4/0	4/4/1	5/3/1	5/4/1	4/3/0

INTERIM STAFF

A second option available to Janet is to depend on the per-diem pool and short-hour nurses. In Janet's facility the per-diem and short-hour nurses receive a 25 percent differential in lieu of fringe benefits. This rate applies to nurses employed to work in a variety of capacities; the choice in many instances is based, however, on the desires of the employee. The per-diem and short-hour nurses are individuals hired to work on an intermittent basis, individuals hired as interim replacements or for temporary work on a predetermined schedule not extending beyond three months, or individuals regularly scheduled to work a predetermined work schedule of less than 20 hours per week. As might be expected, most per-diem/short-hour nurses consider themselves individuals hired to work on an intermittent basis only according to their needs. Consequently the per-diem/short-hour nurse is unavailable for weekend duty approximately 75 percent of the time. In essence the per-diem/short-hour nurse is of no help to Janet.

Such loopholes in contractual agreements have negatively impacted Janet's staffing objectives. But such loopholes have also generated some creative thinking on Janet's part. Although creative thinking alone will not assure balanced staffing immediately, Janet fully recognizes and appreciates the need for long-range planning. Part of Janet's long-range plan is to influence the outcomes of the negotiation process between the hospital administration and the nurses association. Janet and her peer group plan for future staffing needs by designing viable staffing to meet their needs.

Initially the group intended to revise and correct the numerous loopholes in the contractual agreements. Although there was merit in this endeavor, the group soon discovered contractual revisions and corrections would not assure a viable staffing plan. For example, the nursing association recommended redefining the per-diem/short-hour nurse and hiring more individuals in this category. Attempting to establish a commitment from the group redefining the status and role of the per-diem/short-hour nurse was fruitless. Of the 40 nurses comprising the per-diem pool, 75 percent were unavailable for weekend duty and 80 percent were unavailable for night duty. Furthermore, the nursing administration could not approve or disapprove vacation requests or leaves of absence from the per-diem pool individuals; vacations and leaves of absences are benefits granted to part-time and full-time nursing personnel. With per-diem status, personnel waive all benefits and opt for a 25 percent differential in salary. Therefore, the nursing administration had no authority to request, let alone approve, a benefit to which these employees were not entitled.

As a result, the group consensus was that the nursing department no longer needed more individuals on board who were more interested in controlling their own schedules than contributing to the institution's functions. The group determined that the per-diem/short-hour nurse pool was unable to supplement the specific scheduling needs. The hospital needed a group of part-time and full-time individuals willing to work according to a predetermined schedule prepared by the nursing administration. Another subgroup of nurses was developed: float nurses.

Float nurses would be either part-time or full-time employees assigned to one designated shift. Wages and benefits would be the same for these individuals as any other part-time or full-time employee. The unit coordinators would continue to prepare the schedules for their units. These schedules would then be submitted to the staffing coordinator in the nursing administration. The staffing coordinator would be responsible for scheduling the float pool for a tour of duty every other weekend and, where appropriate, during the week, based on the holes in daily staffing plans. In this way the situation that Janet encountered on the weekend of the 7th and 8th (Exhibit 15-1) would be resolved.

Furthermore, a part-time/full-time float pool is cost effective in two ways. First, the wages are 25 percent less than the per diem pool nurses. Second, the schedules are predetermined and based on the needs of the facility. Their reliability and dependability will prevent the overuse of double shifts, overtime, and contracting of registry personnel while simultaneously decreasing burnout among the nursing staff.

OTHER ALTERNATIVES

Job sharing is another viable long-range plan considered by the group. Basically, job sharing would require two consenting employees to coordinate their schedules so that all workdays would be scheduled alternately or opposingly. For example, the schedules of Mary and Karen (Exhibit 15-1) illustrate this point. As the full-time employee, Mary is scheduled to be off Sunday, Wednesday, Monday, and Saturday. Karen, the part-time employee, is scheduled to work on Mary's days off. Both employees may on occasion work similar days, but they are never scheduled *off* on the same days. Should either Mary or Karen wish to revise their schedules, the changes would be agreeable to both employees. If Karen wished to be off on Wednesday the 4th instead of Tuesday the 3rd, Mary would be expected to work as Karen's replacement. Concurrently Mary would be off on Tuesday the 3rd while Karen would work. In this way the basic need of seven-day coverage and the fulfillment of the daily staffing plan are not adversely affected. Furthermore, job sharing of this nature commits the employee to the daily staffing plan, the patients, and the peer group.

Both the part-time/full-time float pool and job-sharing concepts are futuristic plans that Janet's group considers viable. Neither plan will resolve the staffing issues immediately. However, such planning provides hope for better scheduling and staffing and allows Janet to cope with the present.

Although Janet recognizes her weekend staffing shortages, she considers yet another alternative. Maybe she ought to convert two full-time equivalents into three part-time employees. For instance, both Terry's and Cheryl's full-time positions (Exhibit 15-1) could be converted into three 0.6 positions. This would provide Janet with a total of eight RNs, who could be evenly distributed over the weekends. The end result would be that Janet and Mary would be the only remaining full-time RNs. Such a plan would devastate the RN coverage during the weekdays. Therefore, Janet does not consider this plan of action viable. She finds herself in a Catch-22 situation but elects to maintain her staffing pattern, as indicated in Exhibit 15-1.

Janet's final alternative at this time is to schedule the ward clerk to counterbalance the RN shortages. This constitutes a trade-off on Janet's part but will equalize the staffing to a certain degree in terms of numbers of staff and not levels of staff. It would be absurd to schedule the ward clerk for the same weekends in which four RNs are available for duty at the expense of further depleting the staffing on the weekends when only three RNs are available for duty. Hence, Sheila, the ward clerk, is scheduled to work the weekend of the 7th and the 8th. She is scheduled off on those weekdays when there appears to be an abundance of RNs and LVNs (Exhibit 15-1). Even though Janet's master daily staffing plan calls for a ward clerk every day, Janet may elect to replace her with an RN or LVN on certain occasions.

Vacation requests and subsequent approval of those requests can adversely affect the needed daily staffing plan. Granting vacations according to seniority while attempting to stagger leave and thus avoid overlapping vacations will help to minimize the effect of those requests. Other strategies should be incorporated. Once again the weekend staffing cannot be overlooked. Mary may request a two-week vacation. If she requests the vacation to begin on Monday the 2nd and end on Friday the 13th, then the weekend preceding the 2nd and the weekend succeeding the 13th will be included as part of her vacation (Exhibit 15-1). In contrast, Terry may request her vacation for the same time period as Mary. Terry may also assume that the preceding and succeeding weekends are part of her vacation request. This need not be the case; vacations should be granted in accordance with the cyclic scheduling pattern. Thus approving Terry's request would further jeopardize the weekend staffing.

Vacation requests of part-time employees need to be monitored closely. Not only can weekend coverage be adversely affected but weekday coverage can become skeletonlike without close monitoring. For example, as a part-time employee, Joan is eligible for six days of accrued vacation (Exhibit 15-1). With strategic planning on her part, coupled with an oversight by Janet, Joan could conceivably manipulate scheduling to create a two-week vacation. In other words Joan might request the 1st, 5th, 6th, 10th, 11th, and 14th as vacation days and expect her scheduled days off to remain in effect. Approval of this request would result in a two-week vacation whereas approval of the request based on eligible vacation days would result in a total of eight days off. This is not to imply that vacations can never be extended to include scheduled days off. But six-day vacations can be easily converted into two-week vacations—equal to those vacations earned by the full-time employee—if this aspect of staffing is not monitored.

In summary, Janet's situation is a real one, based on the mathematical results of position control. A systematic approach to schedules and staffing will provide nursing administration with an improved logical staffing pattern. In addition, the importance of scheduling according to position control and the daily staffing plan should be noted. Per-diem pools, float pools, job sharing, flexible scheduling, and 10- to 12-hour shifts will have no beneficial effect on staffing patterns without coordinated position control, nor will they have any effect on staffing patterns if scheduling is done in a haphazard manner. The schedule presented in Exhibit 15-1 should be used as a model. Keeping in mind the interplay between position control and scheduling while simultaneously educating staff members to this interplay will increase cooperation among the staff members to adhere to the established guidelines. There will be special requests requiring changes, but staff members may come to appreciate the efforts of nursing administration to maintain staffing coverage in such a manner. Furthermore, staff members can clearly see how their efforts and cooperation can positively impact the goal of the nursing department: patient care.

Chapter 16

Numbers of Staff versus Staff Allocation

OBJECTIVES

Following completion of this chapter the reader will be able to:

- determine productive time expressed in minutes,
- calculate total patient census, total patient acuity, and average patient acuity,
- distribute patient assignments evenly among staff members based on patient acuity versus patient census, and
- allocate levels of staff based on patient acuity.

The process of developing a patient classification system and position control does not begin and end at the unit level. Indeed, decentralization allows assistant directors of nursing and supervisors to delegate certain responsibilities and activities that were once their domain. In the meantime, decentralization allows staff nurses and unit coordinators to develop expertise in areas formerly unknown to them. But mere delegation of the patient classification system and position control to the unit level does not relieve assistant directors of nursing and supervisors of their responsibilities for both processes.

Both the patient classification system and position control must be a coordinated and integrated effort between the nursing units and nursing administration. Unit coordinators assume 24-hour responsibility and accountability for their particular area even though they are not on the premises 24 hours a day. In their absence the assistant directors of nursing and supervisors serve as an extension of the unit coordinator and those responsibilities. Inherent in the responsibilities are an in-depth understanding and appreciation of the patient classification system and a desire to maintain position control. Let us direct our attention to nursing administration and the manner in which the information obtained from the patient classification system is deciphered and interpreted.

PATIENT ACUITY AND CENSUS

Up until this point the total patient acuity reasonably managed by one staff member has not been established. Again simple mathematics and logic are needed. Each tour of duty consists of 8.5 hours. The employee receives payment for 8 hours while the remaining 0.5 hour is an unpaid meal period. The employee receives two 15-minute break periods, thereby reducing the productive time to 7.5 hours. These 7.5 hours represent the absolute maximum productive time in which an employee can possibly deliver patient care.

The productive time is directly related to the relative value unit. [One RVU represents both a minimum amount of time (1 minute) and a maximum amount of time (6 minutes).] Productive time too must be converted into minutes. Multiplying 7.5 hours by 60 minutes can determine productive time expressed in minutes (450 minutes). In other words an employee has a maximum of 450 minutes in one tour of duty to deliver patient care. Therefore, the maximum total acuity that one staff member should be expected to assume is 75, as 75 multiplied by 6 (the maximum amount of time represented by one RVU) yields 450 minutes.

Unit coordinators and charge nurses or their designees are responsible for assessing the acuity of each patient once per shift. The individual acuities ascertained from the patient classification system and incorporated into the kardex are then transcribed onto the daily patient rand (Exhibit 16-1). The total individual acuity is indicated in the upper right-hand corner while any outstanding remarks (IVs, heparin plugs, IV riders, etc.) are indicated in the appropriate box.

From the individual assessments three fluctuating variables are determined: (1) total census, (2) total acuity, and (3) average patient acuity. Total census and total acuity are simply the sum of all patients on the unit and all patient acuities, respectively. The average patient acuity is determined by dividing the total acuity by the total census. For example, Janet's total census is 28 while the total acuity equals 532. Dividing 532 by 28 yields an average patient acuity of 19. These variables are then transcribed onto the unit report, as illustrated by Exhibit 16-2. Total census, total acuity, and average patient acuity are necessary to determine the number of staff needed. Other variables, such as the number of IVs, heparin plugs, and IV riders, become just as important as the unit coordinators and assistant directors attempt to allocate their staff properly.

Both the number of staff and the staff allocation are determined for the most part by the information obtained from the unit report and submitted by the previous shift (i.e., day staffing and allocation are based on the unit report submitted by the night shift; evening staffing and allocation are based on the unit report submitted by the day shift; and night staffing is based on the unit report submitted by the evening shift).

Referring to Janet's daily staffing plan (Chapter 14) will help illustrate the value of total census, total acuity, and average patient acuity. For a census of 28 on the

Exhibit 16-1 Daily Patient Rand

ROOM	NAME	SEX	AGE	DOCTOR	DIAGNOSIS	DAYS	PMS	NOCS
101A	SMITH	F	32	PECK	APPENDICITIS			
101B	" "	F	27	" "	VARICOSE VEINS			
102A	" "	F	44	" "	GANGLION L WRIST			
102B	" "	F	53	" "	R LUNG LESION			
102C	" "	F	73	" "	NASAL FRACTURE			
102D	" "	F	50	" "	L INGUINAL HERNIA			
103A	" "	M	33	" "	CHOLECYSTITIS			
103B	" "	M	37	" "	GASTRIC LESION			
104A	" "	F	67	" "	HEMORRHOIDS			
104B	" "	F	73	" "	FX. R ANKLE			
105A	" "	M	69	" "	CATARACT R EYE			
105B	" "	M	68	" "	DEVIATED SEPTUM			
106A	" "	M	24	" "	GANGLION L WRIST			
106B	" "	M	39	" "	RENAL STONES			
106C	" "	M	55	" "	FX. R ULNA			
106D	" "	M	61	" "	RENAL STONES			
107A	" "	M	65	" "	FX. R TIBIA			
107B	" "	M	45	" "	BOWEL OBSTRUCTION			
108A	" "	M	31	" "	R INGUINAL HERNIA			
108B	" "	M	37	" "	GALLSTONES			
109A	" "	F	77	" "	RENAL STONES			
109B	" "	F	79	" "	APPENDICITIS			
110A	" "	M	84	" "	HAMMER TOES			
110B	" "	M	54	" "	GASTRIC CA			
110C	" "	M	71	" "	FX MANDIBLE			
110D	" "	M	60	" "	CATARACT L EYE			
111A	" "	F	47	" "	FX. L HIP			
111B	" "	F	56	" "	UTERINE TUMOR			

DATE:________

TOTAL CENSUS:________

TOTAL ACUITY:________

AV. ACUITY:________

RN:________

Source: Reprinted with permission of Nursing Department, Doctors Hospital of Pinole, Pinole, California.

Exhibit 16-2 Unit Report

UNIT________ DATE________ DAY________ NURSE________

SHIFT	CENSUS	ACUITY	AVERAGE ACUITY
DAYS			
PMS			
NOCS			

DIFFERENTIAL INFORMATION

SUBJECT	DAYS	PMS	NOCS
INTRAVENOUS FEEDINGS			
HEPARIN PLUGS			
INTRAVENOUS RIDERS			
TRANSFUSIONS			
HYPERALIMENTATION			
HEPARIN DRIPS			
PRE-OP SURGERIES			
POST-OP SURGERIES			
CONFUSED/COMBATIVE PTS.			
ISOLATIONS			

Source: Reprinted with permission of Nursing Department, Doctors Hospital of Pinole, Pinole, California.

day shift Janet requested eight staff members: one unit coordinator, one ward clerk, three RNs, and three LVNs/LPNs. The unit coordinator and the ward clerk do not participate in direct patient care. Therefore, six staff members are available to deliver patient care. Janet wanted to limit the total acuity per staff member to a maximum of 75. Without a patient classification system, Janet might merely distribute the assignment by attempting to divide the number of patients evenly among the staff. Such an assignment appears in Table 16-1.

The pitfalls of this traditional method of distributing patient assignments have disappeared with the advent of patient classification systems. The preceding assignment does not define patient acuity and intensity; it simply provides a fairly evenly distributed patient assignment to the naked eye. By determining average patient acuity and the acuity range, unit coordinators, assistant directors of

Table 16-1 Patient Assignment Based on Census

Nurse A	*Nurse B*	*Nurse C*	*Nurse D*	*Nurse E*	*Nurse F*
102A	101A	104A	106A	111A	110A
102B	101B	104B	106B	111B	110B
102C	103B	107A	106C	108A	110C
102D	105A	107B	106D	108B	110D
103A	105B	109A	109B		

nursing, and supervisors are able to staff according to patient needs and therefore justify both positive and negative variances from Janet's daily staffing plan. Comparing and contrasting the unit reports to the daily schedule will help illustrate this process.

Reviewing Unit Reports

As Janet reports to work on Tuesday, October 3, she reviews the unit report submitted by the night shift. The census is 28, the acuity is 532, and the average patient acuity is 19. Nine staff members are available to work according to the corresponding schedule (Exhibit 15-1). In terms of the budget and position control (Table 14-10), only eight staff members should be utilized for a census of 28. To decrease her staff to eight Janet may float either the ward clerk or a licensed staff member. If she floats the ward clerk, the patient/staff ratio will not be affected but the secretarial responsibilities for the unit may go by the wayside. On the other hand, floating a licensed staff member will alter the patient/staff ratio. Floating a licensed staff member provides Janet with six staff members to deliver patient care. Janet may elect to distribute the patients as shown in Table 16-2.

The total acuities far exceed the desired acuity. Even if Janet elected to distribute the patient assignments based on total census, as in the past, coupled with the present acuity system, she would discover gross imbalances in the assignment (Table 16-3). Immediately Janet is alerted to the fact that nurse D's

Table 16-2 Patient Assignment Based on Budget and Position Control

	Nurse A		*Nurse B*		*Nurse C*		*Nurse D*		*Nurse E*		*Nurse F*	
	Pat.	Ac.	Pat.	Ac.	Pat.	Ac.	Pat.	Ac.	Pat.	Ac.	Pat.	Ac.
	102A	15	101A	17	104B	23	106A	30	111A	28	109B	20
	102B	21	101B	12	105B	20	106B	18	111B	19	110A	22
	102C	12	103A	22	107A	17	106C	14	108A	16	110B	16
	102D	23	104A	24	107B	16	106D	20	108B	25	110C	12
	103B	18	105A	18	109A	17					110D	17
Total		89		93		93		82		88		87

Table 16-3 Patient Assignment Based on Census and Respective Acuities

Nurse A		Nurse B		Nurse C		Nurse D		Nurse E		Nurse F	
Pat.	Ac.	Pat.	Ac.	Pat.	Ac.	Pat.	Ac.	Pat.	Ac.	Pat.	Ac.
102A	15	101A	17	104A	24	106A	30	108A	16	110A	22
102B	21	101B	12	104B	23	106B	18	108B	25	110B	16
102C	12	103B	18	107A	17	106C	14	111A	28	110C	12
102D	23	105A	18	107B	16	106D	20	111B	19	110D	17
103A	22	105B	20	109A	17	109B	20				
Total	93		85		97		102		88		67

Average Patient Acuity = 19

assignment (102) far outweighs nurse F's assignment (67). Individual acuities in this case become unimportant because the average patient acuity will ultimately define the acuity range assumed by staff members. The number of patients per staff member as well as the average patient acuity (19) remains the same with both assignments. Because some staff members will assume responsibility for 4 patients while other staff members will assume responsibility for 5 patients, Janet is able to determine the acuity range. Multiplying the average patient acuity (19) by the minimum and maximum number of patients assigned to staff members (4 and 5, respectively) will yield the acuity range (76 to 95).

This range represents an unrealistic acuity for any one staff member to absorb and maintain quality patient care. The maximum total acuity per staff member should not and cannot exceed 75 as one eight-hour tour of duty does not provide enough minutes to absorb a higher acuity. On the other hand an average patient acuity of 15 will yield an acuity range of 60 to 75 (Table 16-4), which complements Janet's daily staffing plan well.

Table 16-4 Patient Assignment Based on Census and Average Patient Acuity of 15

Nurse A		Nurse B		Nurse C		Nurse D		Nurse E		Nurse F	
Pat.	Ac.	Pat.	Ac.	Pat.	Ac.	Pat.	Ac.	Pat.	Ac.	Pat.	Ac.
102A	12	101A	15	104A	20	106A	21	108A	16	110A	22
102B	15	101B	12	104B	16	106B	12	108B	15	110B	16
102C	12	103B	14	107A	16	106C	12	111A	21	110C	12
102D	20	105A	15	107B	10	106D	10	111B	14	110D	17
103A	14	105B	17	109A	10	109B	14				
Total	73		73		72		69		66		67

Any average patient acuity exceeding 15, given a census of 28, should immediately alert the unit coordinators, the assistant directors of nursing, and the supervisors that a staffing increase is warranted and justified. By providing one additional staff member above budget and position control Janet is able to adjust the acuity range (Table 16-5). The patient/staff ratio theoretically becomes 4 to 1 while the acuity range becomes a constant 76. A total acuity of 76 is far more reasonable than one of 95. Although a total acuity of 76 appears more reasonable than one of 95, 76 is far from perfect. In fact, it will take two additional nurses above budget and position control to decrease the acuity range so that it coincides with the guidelines (Table 16-6).

Adjusting the Acuity Range

By adding two staff members, some staff members will assume responsibility for three patients while others will assume responsibility for four patients. Again, multiplying the average patient acuity (19) by 3 and 4 will yield the adjusted acuity range (57 to 76). There is no doubt that Janet will find this acuity range the most reasonable. If she elected to staff her unit with only one additional nurse as opposed to two, then the nurses would most likely experience high stress and the

Table 16-5 Patient Assignment Based on Census of 28, with 1 Additional Staff Member, and Average Patient Acuity of 19

	Nurse A		*Nurse B*		*Nurse C*		*Nurse D*		*Nurse E*		*Nurse F*		*Nurse G*	
	Pat.	*Ac.*	*Pat.*	*Ac.*	*Pat.*	*Ac.*	*Pat.*	*Ac.*	*Pat.*	*Ac.*	*Pat.*	*Ac.*	*Pat.*	*Ac.*
	101A	17	102C	12	103A	22	101B	12	106B	18	106D	20	109B	20
	102A	15	104A	24	103B	18	105A	18	106C	14	109A	17	110B	16
	102B	21	104B	23	105B	20	106A	30	108B	25	110A	22	110C	12
	102C	23	107A	17	107B	16	108A	16	111B	19	110D	17	111A	28
		—		—		—		—		—		—		—
Total		76		76		76		76		76		76		76

Table 16-6 Patient Assignment Based on Census of 28, with 2 Additional Staff Members, and Average Patient Acuity of 19

	Nurse A		*Nurse B*		*Nurse C*		*Nurse D*		*Nurse E*		*Nurse F*		*Nurse G*		*Nurse H*	
	Pat.	Ac.	Pat.	Ac.	Pat.	Ac.	Pat.	Ac.	Pat.	Ac.	Pat.	Ac.	Pat.	Ac.	Pat.	Ac.
	102A	15	101A	17	104A	24	101B	12	106A	30	106D	20	109B	20	110A	22
	102B	21	102D	23	104B	23	103A	22	106B	18	108A	16	111A	28	110B	16
	102C	12	107A	16	105A	18	103B	18	106C	14	108B	25	111B	19	110C	12
	109A	17	107B	17			105B	20							110D	17
		—		—		—		—		—		—		—		—
Total		65		73		65		72		62		61		67		67

patients, inadequate care. An acuity range that begins and ends at 76, already above the desired norm of 75, leaves no room to accommodate the unpredictable and the intangibles not included in the kardex or patient classification system (admitting patients, discharging patients, cardiac arrests, etc.). Staffing should not focus on the unpredictable or the intangibles, but should be based on the available time frame (450 minutes).

Conversely, extremely low average patient acuities affect the number of staff needed proportionally. Perhaps the average patient acuity for a census of 28 is only 10 (Table 16-7). With Janet's daily staffing plan of six staff members delivering direct patient care, an average patient acuity of 10 alters the acuity range per staff member to 40 to 50.

Because the average patient acuity is 10, maybe five staff members could easily manage patient care as opposed to the designated six staff members. Distributing the patient assignment among five staff members appears in Table 16-8.

Table 16-7 Patient Assignment Based on Census of 28 and Average Patient Acuity of 10

	Nurse A		*Nurse B*		*Nurse C*		*Nurse D*		*Nurse E*		*Nurse F*	
	Pat.	Ac.	Pat.	Ac.	Pat.	Ac.	Pat.	Ac.	Pat.	Ac.	Pat.	Ac.
	101A	13	102A	15	104B	8	107A	8	109B	12	106C	10
	101B	14	102B	6	105B	10	107B	14	110A	14	106D	13
	103A	10	102C	11	106A	18	108A	10	110B	10	111A	13
	103B	8	102D	5	106B	10	108B	6	110C	7	111B	10
	105A	5	104A	7			109A	7	110D	6		
Total		50		44		46		45		49		46

Table 16-8 Patient Assignment Based on Census of 28, Decreasing by 1 Staff Member, and Average Patient Acuity of 10

	Nurse A		*Nurse B*		*Nurse C*		*Nurse D*		*Nurse E*	
	Pat.	Ac.	Pat.	Ac.	Pat.	Ac.	Pat.	Ac.	Pat	Ac.
	101A	13	102A	15	104B	8	106C	10	107A	8
	101B	14	102B	6	106A	18	106D	13	110A	14
	103A	10	102C	11	106B	10	109A	7	110B	10
	103B	8	102D	5	107B	14	109B	12	110C	7
	105A	5	104A	7	108B	6	111A	13	110D	6
	105B	10	108A	10					111B	10
Total		60		54		56		55		55

Such an assignment would redefine the acuity range. Decreasing the number of staff by one merely increases the acuity range from 40–50 to 50–60, a range within the guidelines of the staffing system.

Janet may also consider decreasing the staff by two staff members (Table 16-9). In this case the patient/staff ratio becomes 7 to 1 while the acuity range becomes a constant 70. Therefore Janet has the option to decrease the number of staff not only by one nurse but also by two nurses. This option becomes extremely important when Janet must flex her staffing to accommodate low-census, high-acuity patients, as discussed in Chapter 14. The rule of thumb should be to decrease the staff when appropriate; saving dollars and cents during these periods will allow greater flexibility in times of need.

Adjusting the number of staff on a particular unit to coincide with the most appropriate and reasonable acuity range alone will not assure quality patient care. According to nursing policy, patient care will be delivered by a licensed professional staff whenever possible. This licensed professional staff, consisting of registered nurses and licensed vocational nurses/licensed practical nurses, will be allocated according to patient care needs. As patient census and acuity fluctuate, so too will the number and type of staff needed to deliver quality patient care. However, despite the unpredictable fluctuations, a minimum number of RNs is necessary to manage these uncontrollable circumstances safely and efficiently. Minimum guidelines for the medical/surgical units are given in Table 16-10.

These guidelines are based on input from unit coordinators and staff members. Attempting to coordinate patient care on 1 South for 28 patients on the day shift with less than three RNs proved devastating. Experience demonstrated that staffing with two RNs was, in essence, nothing more than staffing by the team leading concept. One RN would be assigned to the desk, while the other RN would be assigned the overall responsibility for the 28 patients. Excessive overtime, as

Table 16-9 Patient Assignment Based on Census of 28, Decreasing by 2 Staff Members, and Average Patient Acuity of 10

	Nurse A		*Nurse B*		*Nurse C*		*Nurse D*	
	Pat.	Ac.	Pat.	Ac.	Pat.	Ac.	Pat.	Ac.
	101A	13	102A	15	104B	8	104A	7
	101B	14	102B	6	106A	18	106C	10
	103A	10	102C	11	106B	10	109A	7
	103B	8	102D	5	107A	8	109B	12
	105A	5	106D	13	107B	14	110A	14
	105B	10	108A	10	108B	6	110C	7
	110B	10	111B	10	110D	6	111A	13
Total		70		70		70		70

Table 16-10 Minimum Number of Nurses for Medical/Surgical Units

Unit	*Days*	*PMs*	*NOCs*	*Bed Capacity*	*Projected Daily Census*
1 S	3	3	2	34	28
1 N	3	3	2	24	18
2 S	3	3	2	28	18
2 N	2	2	1	16	14

well as justified fatigue, irritability, and frustration, were the byproducts of this particular staffing pattern. Staffing with at least three RNs on a day-to-day basis markedly decreased these hazards. However, on certain occasions, three RNs were not enough to decrease overtime, fatigue, irritability and frustration. Basically, then, how do unit coordinators, assistant directors of nursing, and supervisors appropriately allocate their staff? How do they know the number of RNs needed versus the number of LVNs/LPNs needed?

DIFFERENTIAL INFORMATION

Differential information (see Exhibit 16-2) will help justify fluctuating RN/LVN ratios. Granted, the RN and LVN staff have become more harmonious in terms of technical skills. The LVN staff have been inserviced and educated to both drug administration and IV therapy. They can insert foley catheters, monitor enteral nutrition, change dressings, irrigate nasal gastric tubes, change colostomy bags, administer enemas, empty bedpans, give bed baths—and all for less money. Therefore, why is there concern about RN/LVN ratios? Why shouldn't the unit establish a baseline minimum of RNs needed and supplement with LVNs? But a definite line of demarcation exists between these two professional groups. This line of demarcation becomes defined by the first six subjects of differential information.

Just as unit coordinators and charge nurses are responsible for assessing patient acuities once per shift, they are responsible for completing the differential information once per shift. Like individual acuities, the differential information is obtained from the daily patient rand (Exhibit 16-1). However, the patient kardex and staff members must be utilized to obtain some of this information. For instance, Janet has indicated on the daily patient rand that five patients have IVs while six patients have heparin plugs. To determine the number of IV riders she must either refer to the patient kardex and count the number of IV riders to be administered on her shift or, better yet, ask her staff members for the IV rider count, because they are the ones administering the medications. The quickest way to obtain the number of IV riders is simply to obtain the facts from the staff members. As Janet determines the number of intravenous feedings, heparin plugs, IV riders, transfusions, etc., she enters the figures on the unit report (Exhibit 16-2).

According to hospital policy LVNs may start, superimpose, and maintain intravenous solutions. This policy may appear rather broad but in reality it is extremely limiting because LVNs may start, superimpose, and maintain only those IV solutions containing nutrients, vitamins, and minerals—and only within certain dosages. Consequently, heparin plugs requiring daily heparin irrigations, intravenous antibiotics piggybacked via a heparin plug or parenteral IV, hyperalimentation containing insulin, and heparin drips must be managed by a registered nurse although the LVN may manage a plain IV of dextrose and water and a blood transfusion. Hence, the figures obtained will markedly influence the type of staff needed and warranted. Let us compare Janet's daily schedule with the unit report over a three-day period to demonstrate how the differential information can affect staffing patterns.

Availability of Staff

To begin, the availability for the nursing staff must be determined. Does the daily schedule (Exhibit 15-1) reflect Janet's daily staffing plan (Exhibit 14-3)? As Janet's schedule indicates, five RNs, four LVNs, and one ward clerk are scheduled to work on Monday, October 2; five RNs, three LVNs, and one ward clerk are scheduled to work on Tuesday, October 3; and five RNs, four LVNs, and one ward clerk are scheduled to work on Wednesday, October 4. Janet's daily schedule reflects her daily staffing plan of eight staff members. In fact, the schedule reflects more staff than required. The corresponding unit report for 1 South for the day shift indicates the data in Table 16-11.

When comparing the actual census to the budgeted number of staff (Table 14-10), Janet will discover that for each respective day too many staff members are scheduled. However, before Janet readjusts staffing, she must consider patient acuities.

Considering Patient Acuities

By quickly scanning the unit reports, Janet is able to determine that the average patient acuity on October 3 and 4 far exceeds the desired acuity of 15 compared to the average patient acuity on October 2. Furthermore, the number of IVs, heparin plugs, and IV riders on October 3 and 4 are far greater than those of October 2. In essence Janet faces two dilemmas. On October 2 her concern is merely the number of staff members because the average patient acuity is within the norm, while on October 3 and 4 she is dealing with both the number of staff and the allocation of staff.

Table 16-11 Unit Report Data

Date	*Census*	*Acuity*	*Average Acuity*
Oct. 2	29	432	14.9
Oct. 3	28	532	19.0
Oct. 4	18	375	20.8

	Differential Information		
Subject	*Oct. 2*	*Oct. 3*	*Oct. 4*
Intravenous feedings	2	5	6
Heparin plugs	1	6	6
IV riders	4	12	10
Transfusions	-	1	2
Hyperalimentation	-	1	1
Heparin drips	-	1	1
Preop surgeries	3	1	4
Postop surgeries	3	3	1
Confused/combative pts.	-	-	-
Isolations	-	-	-

Essentially, from a budget perspective Janet may utilize 8.11 (Table 14-10) staff members on the day shift. Three of the 8 staff members must be RNs according to the minimum guidelines (Table 16-10). The remaining staff members will most likely be 4 LVNs and 1 ward clerk, thereby affording Janet a total of 6 licensed individuals to deliver direct patient care. The activity involved with two IVs, one heparin plug, and four IV riders does not warrant an extra RN; 2 RNs can safely and efficiently manage this workload. Utilizing this RN/LVN ratio will establish an acuity range of 59.6 to 74.5, which each staff member will have to absorb. Because Janet has 10 staff members scheduled to work and can reasonably manage the patient care with 8 staff members, 2 staff members (RNs) may be allocated elsewhere in the hospital.

The picture is drastically different on October 3 and 4. The high average patient acuities justify additional staff members. The unit report indicates intense activity related to IVs, heparin plugs, hyperalimentation, etc. The information provides Janet with the insight necessary to determine the type of additional staff needed. The rather limiting IV policy under which LVNs must function aids Janet in her decision-making process. In other words Janet chooses an RN as the additional staff member because LVNs cannot heparinize heparin plugs, administer IV antibiotics, or manage hyperalimentation and heparin drips. Consequently it would not boost patient care to enlist the services of an LVN when the differential information indicates intense activity in areas where LVNs should not assume responsibility.

Hence, on October 3 Janet elects to staff at least four RNs and four LVNs to maintain an appropriate acuity range (57 to 76) in addition to herself and the ward clerk. In contrast on October 4 Janet allocates the ward clerk to another unit because the total census is 18 and Janet feels that she can adequately function in both capacities. The average patient acuity calls for six staff members to deliver patient care if an appropriate acuity range is to be determined (62.4). Once again the intense activity associated with parenteral fluids makes it necessary for Janet to staff the unit with at least four RNs delivering direct patient care.

REPORTS FROM THE UNIT

Once the unit reports have been completed, the information must be transmitted to the assistant directors of nursing and the relief supervisors. The manner in which the assistant directors and relief supervisors retrieve this information may vary from person to person and from day to day. Sometimes the information is relayed via the telephone, and the assistant director and relief supervisor or secretary transcribe the information onto the nursing office report (Exhibit 16-3). At other times the assistant director and relief supervisor may elect to retrieve the information in person from the unit coordinator and transcribe the information at that time. In either case the communication must take place for the assistant director/relief supervisor to serve in the absence of the unit coordinators and maintain staffing throughout the hospital.

Although the unit coordinators have an in-depth understanding and clear picture of their units, they do not have the same understanding and picture of the entire hospital. Janet does not know the total census, total acuity, and average patient acuity of all the nursing units. In addition, she is unaware of the staffing patterns and the availability of staff in other areas of the hospital. The information contained in the nursing office report cannot and will not be interpreted from different perspectives. All nursing managers know that the average patient acuity assumed by any one individual cannot exceed 75. All nursing managers know that intense activity surrounding parenteral fluids indicates the need for an extra RN. Finally, all nursing managers know the minimum number of RNs needed on each shift each day. As a result, Janet, the assistant director, and relief supervisor know the staffing needs for 1 South. However, only the assistant director and relief supervisor are capable of allocating the staff for they are the ones who know the needs of all the nursing units. In other words, who floats to Janet's unit in the event she needs an additional staff member is beyond her control. It becomes the responsibility of the assistant director and relief supervisor to assign the staff according to patient care needs.

Assistant directors and relief supervisors, because they are responsible for staffing, share budgetary responsibilities also. Because they staff according to the

Exhibit 16-3 Nursing Office Report

DATE: ________ SHIFT: ________ A.D.O.N. ________

	ONE SOUTH	ONE NORTH	TWO SOUTH	TWO NORTH
TOTAL CENSUS				
TOTAL ACUITY				
AVERAGE PATIENT ACUITY				
ACUITY RANGE				
INTRAVENOUS FEEDINGS				
HEPARIN PLUGS				
INTRAVENOUS RIDERS				
TRANSFUSIONS				
HYPERALIMENTATION				
HEPARIN DRIPS				
PRE-OP SURGERIES				
POST-OP SURGERIES				
CONFUSED PATIENTS				
ISOLATIONS				

Source: Reprinted with permission of Nursing Department, Doctors Hospital of Pinole, Pinole, California.

information contained in the nursing office report they must assume that the information is accurate and correct. Should one become suspicious of the accuracy and correctness of the information, the nursing office report provides the assistant director and relief supervisor a manner in which to audit charts. When total acuities remain stagnant as well as individual acuities, perhaps it is time for the assistant director and relief supervisor to conduct such an audit. By comparing the information marked on the individual's kardex with the patient's chart, one is able to determine the accuracy of the patient classification system and ultimately the nursing office report. For example, the kardex may indicate that the patient requires a complete bed bath while the nursing notes state that a shower was taken. In this case the entire acuity is altered, which affects the total acuity in the long run.

Periodic audits of this nature can assure accuracy with the patient classification system. Some errors are truly innocent oversights, but consistent errors are inexcusable. It behooves the unit coordinators and charge nurses to assess the patients accurately. Underestimating the care that a patient requires results in staffing shortages, but overestimating the care may result in too much staff, thereby affecting costs. If a particular unit consistently overestimates the care that a patient requires and the assistant director and relief supervisor are suspicious of the overestimation, then the assistant director and relief supervisor may elect to staff only according to the census. On the other hand audits performed by the assistant director and relief supervisor will keep them in touch with acute nursing care and not lose sight of the type of care demanded by the physician and warranted by the patient. In this way all nursing managers may appreciate the patient classification system and the staffing patterns defined by it.

Chapter 17

Interpreting a Department Budget as an Integral Part of a Nurse Staffing System

OBJECTIVES

Following completion of this chapter the reader will be able to:

- relate the impact of nursing managers on their units' budget,
- understand the nursing managers' need for being able to interpret their unit budget,
- list the three qualities of a department budget,
- define *unit cost*,
- list the three reports that a nursing manager needs to understand,
- describe how each report should be utilized and interpreted, and
- complete successfully the self-quiz, Appendix 17-A.

When a nursing administrator hires unit managers, one of the objectives in the job description should be that the manager assumes the responsibility for assuring that patients receive quality comprehensive nursing care in the most cost-effective method available. Today, more than ever before, a nursing administrator (director of nursing) looks for nursing unit managers with experience in fiscal management and expects them to be able to interpret and manage sensibly the fiscal affairs of their units as well as manage the patient care directly related to their units. The great expectations that nursing administrators have placed on nursing managers are dramatically opposed to the training that most RNs have received as well as the different priorities essential for most of these nursing managers. As some nursing managers have been known to express, ''If I had wanted to compute operating and capital budgets, I would have become an accountant.''

Nursing administrators need to work closely with their managers, taking the time to teach them and help them, reinforcing as necessary, until they have grasped the concepts that are expected of them to be able to interpret, monitor, and manage sensibly. If nursing managers are the least bit insecure in matters of a fiscal nature, it is up to the supervisor, usually the nursing administrator, to teach, guide, and help the nurse managers to feel secure, while at the same time allowing the managers to develop the self-confidence needed to deal with the new images of the role, that of financial manager of the unit. If this is not accomplished in a timely and supportive manner, nursing administrators may find themselves with high turnover rates in nursing managers.

On the other hand fiscal accountability should remain with the nursing managers. In an age when cost accountability is a reality to managers, the administrator's withholding fiscal accountability from them and accepting complete responsibility only delay the learning process for the nursing manager. As an effective manager and leader, it becomes the responsibility and challenge of the administrator to develop the subordinates' fiscal expertise and to delegate this fiscal responsibility to them when they are ready to assume it.

Placing an importance on budgets and financial management seems to contradict every reason why people became nurses. Most people initially became nurses in order to care for the sick and injured. Regardless of how dramatic this may sound, how many went into nursing desiring to hold nursing management positions? But times have changed and health care has changed; despite the distaste that most nurses may have for the budgetary process and fiscal management, the complex world of mathematics has seeped its way into nursing's already multifaceted jobs.

Many nursing managers lack academic preparation in the area of fiscal management as well as the ability to verbalize logical and realistic facts that justify variations in a unit's budget. While the academic preparation may be lacking in a nursing manager's background, nursing managers of the 1980s find that they must be prepared, knowledgeable, and credible in the area of fiscal management. In order to secure the ears of the financial controller and hospital administrator, a nursing manager must be able to talk on the language level of these two individuals when it comes to matters of money. Leaders in continuing education have begun marketing to these needs and are at last flooding the nursing management conferences with pertinent lectures, seminars, and workshops designed to prepare nursing managers more adequately to be at least skilled in the basics and application of financial management as it pertains to a department of nursing.

Nursing managers should take advantage of these types of programs in order to educate themselves in the area of fiscal management and improve their understanding, thereby establishing credibility with the financial officers. If attendance at workshops, seminars, and lectures is not an attainable goal in the nursing managers' institution from a cost containment standpoint, individuals should seek out peers or perhaps secure the resources of a sympathetic controller rather than operate in the dark and feel frustrated about this important aspect of a manager's position.

Through decentralization of the nursing department the power and authority for the control and management of the nursing unit's dollars are delegated to the unit manager. The sooner unit managers realize the dramatic impact of this authority role on the total operation of each unit and overall hospital functions, the quicker they will want to be heard, acknowledged, and respected for what they may be able to contribute toward the benefit of both their department and the entire facility.

QUALITIES OF A DEPARTMENTAL BUDGET

Of paramount importance is that the nursing manager understand three qualities of a department's budget:

1. the budget as a financial plan
2. the budget as a management tool
3. the budget as a forecast

The Budget as a Financial Plan

The nursing department's budget is a comprehensive financial plan based on anticipated outputs and predetermined hospital goals expressed in terms of revenue dollars and expense dollars. The department's budget becomes an operational plan that summarizes the actual and anticipated activities of each nursing unit whereby the manager can discuss a plan of action with the financial controller or communicate it to the nursing staff.

The Budget as a Management Tool

Through decentralization each nursing manager is given the responsibility to coordinate the unit and its resources. Because the budget is also a management tool, the manager must be able to correlate the information provided in the budget data in order to balance resources and achieve the institution's financial objectives, that is, gross profit.

When looking at one's individual nursing unit budget on a monthly basis, the conscientious manager can initiate a specific plan to organize and control unit operations.

The Budget as a Forecast

The nursing department projects an overall forecast of the quality and cost of services and the amount and source of revenue for the department. It is a basic plan showing all revenue and all expenses necessary to operate the entire nursing department as well as each individual unit. A nursing unit budget is based on the analysis of performance statistics and is adjusted for anticipated operations.

Patient days are estimated and based on historical trend, new physicians expected to join the medical staff, expanded patient population, increased clients from the aging population, and anticipated new services. New services mean that if the hospital should decide to create, to organize, or even just to support a local sports medicine program, this would concurrently increase the number of orthopedic cases referred to the hospital through physicians on staff at the sports medicine clinic, who would probably practice in the local hospitals. The primary objective of a budget then is to monitor and guide the financial affairs of the hospital in order to accomplish the hospital's goals.[1]

Nursing managers determine labor and staffing. By using the budget as a forecast, the nursing manager requests additional staff or limits staff in direct proportion with the patient census. Likewise, the manager increases inventory or modifies ordering of supplies as the patient census varies. The budget sets standards measured as per-unit cost. This is a particularly important key item to monitor in that once the unit cost has been determined, the manager must work within its limits. For example, with med-surg nursing, the unit of measure is hours per patient day. Therefore, the unit of cost per unit of measure tells the nursing manager of a med-surg unit how much it should cost (the unit of cost in dollars) to take care of the patient (the unit of measure in patient days). The budget will state:

$$X \text{ patients} = Y \text{ dollars' worth of nursing care}$$

Another example is the surgery department. In surgery the unit of measure is the number of cases. The critical factor for the unit manager to monitor is the unit of cost (dollars) per unit of measure (cases). Likewise in the emergency department the unit of measure is the number of patient visits. The critical factor for the unit manager to monitor is the unit of cost (dollars) per unit of measure (patient visits); in the central service department, where the unit of measure is the number of line items filled or distributed out to patients, the manager must monitor the unit of cost (dollars) per unit of measure (items distributed). Table 17-1 lists hospital departments and shows monthly units of measure commonly used.

If a nursing unit manager can learn to monitor the cost per unit of measure, the manager can have a tremendous effect on the overall performance of the unit, certainly in terms of dollars and, as a nurse expert in terms of management and patient care. The cost per unit of measure can always reflect directly how the department functions with what has been allotted in the budget.

To summarize, the nursing department's annual budget is a comprehensive financial plan, a management tool, and a forecast, all of which should be compiled to meet the overall goals of the hospital. The budget provides the basis for management control, sets standards for performance, and enables actual and planned performance to be assessed and controlled. Major variances from the budget should then be promptly analyzed to determine if the established budget is unrealistic or if adjusted cost control measures should be implemented.

Table 17-1 Hospital Departments and Monthly Unit of Measure

Department	*Unit of Measure*
Administration	# of pt. days
Business office	# of pt. days
Cardiology	# of procedures
Dietary	# of meals served
Plant operations/maintenance, engineering	square footage of plant/facility
Housekeeping	square footage of plant/facility
Laboratory	# of procedures
Medical records	# of admissions[a]
Nursing units:	
Med-surg	# of pt. days/nursing units
ICU-CCU, etc.	# of pt. days per ICU-CCU
Central service	# of line items filled
Emergency	# of pt. visits
G.I. lab	# of procedures
O.P.S.U.	# of cases
Surgery	# of cases
U.R./D.P.	# of pt. days
Personnel	# of pt. days
Pharmacy	# of prescriptions filled
Physical therapy	# of procedures/treatments
Purchasing	# of pt. days
Respiratory therapy	# of procedures
X-Ray	# of procedures

[a]In some facilities the medical records department may use the number of discharges as the monthly unit of measure.

DEPARTMENT REPORTS

A variety of reports produced periodically in every facility can give a manager valuable departmental information. The information on these reports enables a manager to evaluate performance on the unit and determine expenses compared to budget. While each facility may vary in the type and number of reports generated for use by the nursing managers, every nursing manager ought to be familiar with, receive, and review three financial reports on a regular basis. In most cases, these three monthly reports provide the manager with needed valuable information. These three reports are:

1. labor hours report,
2. operating statement, and
3. expense report.

While facilities may vary in what they choose to title these reports, nursing managers should have access and responsibility for interpreting and monitoring their departments' budget activity reports. Table 17-2 describes the title, general purpose, and key indicators for the appropriate use and frequency of each report.

Labor Hours Report

Each hospital facility has some mechanism for determining and recording total hours worked. Each facility should also have a mechanism for differentiating productive and nonproductive hours worked in a facility in addition to a specific department. The labor hours report for a nursing unit, for instance, should show productive nursing hours as well as nonproductive hours.

In order to interpret this report accurately, one must understand that productive nursing hours are defined as hours spent for direct patient care, that is, hours spent hands-on, actually delivering patient care. The categories of productive nursing hours are:

- regular nursing hours (scheduled hours),
- overtime hours,
- call-back hours, and
- contract hours (registry).

Table 17-2 Monthly Financial Reports for Nursing Department Managers

Table	*Title*	*Purpose*	*Key Indicator/Use*			*Frequency*
17-3	Labor hours report	Shows productive hours per patient day (nursing care hours)	Hours Worked Per Patient Days	=	Regular Hours + Overtime + Callback + Contract Labor ÷ Patient Days	Every pay period
17-4	Operating statement	Summary of department's performance	Gross Profit	=	Revenue − Expenses	Monthly
17-5	Expense report	Shows all bills paid by hospital for monthly expenses of department	Used to identify expenses			Monthly

Productive nursing hours can be abbreviated in the following equation:

regular hours + overtime hours + callback hours + contract hours
= productive nursing hours

Nonproductive nursing hours are defined as the hours spent in areas other than those directly related to patient care. The following examples may be grouped along with the category of nonproductive nursing hours:

- inservice
- orientation
- holiday
- vacation
- sick time
- continuing education tıme
- funeral leave
- jury duty
- standby

Facilities may vary in grouping additional areas of nonproductive nursing time depending on the benefits provided by the facility either according to hospital policy or through contract agreements.

Nonproductive nursing hours are still paid to the employee but are not directly related to hands-on patient care. Some nonproductive hours include benefits such as vacation, holidays, and sick pay. Some of these nonproductive nursing hours can be prescheduled and predetermined. Examples of nonproductive nursing hours that can be prescheduled or predetermined on a fairly accurate basis are:

- vacation
- holiday
- inservice
- orientation
- continuing education hours
- standby.

A number of nonproductive nursing hours cannot be predetermined or prescheduled. Examples of these are:

- sick time
- funeral leave
- jury duty

In other words a simple way to remember the difference between productive and nonproductive nursing hours is that productive hours are:

- any hours actually worked,
- hours previously determined, and
- in most cases scheduled hours directly related to patient care.

While nonproductive hours may still be hours worked, they are *not* related to direct patient care. However, they *are* hours paid. On the other hand nonproductive hours can include hours paid as benefits but not worked.

To determine the nursing hours per patient day, the nurse manager totals the number of productive nursing hours worked and divides this figure by the number of patient days recorded in that accounting period of time. For example, in Table 17-3, there was a total of 1,959 productive nursing hours. If this accounting period showed 349 patient days, the nursing hours per patient day would be 5.72. This is determined in the following manner:

1,999 hours ÷ 349 patient days = 5.72 nursing hours per patient day

The total number of hours paid equals the number of hours worked (productive hours) plus all other hours paid, such as inservice, orientation, vacation, holiday, sick time, jury duty, funeral leave, and educational leave (nonproductive hours).

Also reflected in a labor hours analysis report should be the actual worked and paid FTEs. The total number of full-time equivalents worked is determined by dividing the total number of hours worked by 80, the number of hours in an accounting period. Usually an accounting period is two weeks in length; a full-time employee would work 80 hours during two weeks (40 hours a week). The paid FTEs indicate all the full-time equivalents, both productive and nonproductive, that were charged to the department during the particular accounting period (Table 17-3).

Table 17-3 Labor Hours Report

Town and Country Hospital
Department: 1 South—Medical-Surgical
(2-week period)

Productive Hours				*Nonproductive Hours*				
Regular Hours	*Over-Time*	*Contract Labor*	*Hours Worked*	*Inservice*	*Other (Vacation, Holiday Sick Benefits)*	*Total Hours Paid*	*FTE Worked*	*FTE Paid*
1,924.5	34.5	40.0	1,999.0	99.0	324.5	2,422.5	24.78	30.28

Operating Statement

The monthly operating statement summarizes a given department's financial performance, which will reflect actual unit operations. The key indicator on this report is:

$$\text{gross profit} = \text{revenue} - \text{expenses}$$

Table 17-4 helps understand fully the following discussion of the items that appear on the monthly operating statement.

Unit of Measure: Patient Days. This figure represents the total number of patient days recorded for the month in review. In Table 17-4 this figure represents the combined total of all medical-surgical (med-surg) units. Table 17-4 shows 2,269 med-surg patient days during this month.

Total Revenue. Total revenue refers to the total number of dollars generated through patient room charges of those 2,269 patients. The total revenue on the example in Table 17-4 is \$646,665 (2,269 × \$285 = \$646,665).

Regular Salaries and Wages (with Overtime). This figure refers to the total amount of dollars spent on salaries and wages including the overtime hours (paid at a regular rate) to all nursing staff who worked on the medical-surgical units during this month. In Table 17-4 regular salaries and wages with overtime total \$135,309.

Contract. This represents the amount of dollars spent for contract labor from registry services during the month. In Table 17-4 this amounts to \$1,760. The reader can further break this figure down as to the actual number of hours this represents if the reader knows that the rate is \$22 an hour for an RN. Therefore, if \$1,760 were spent on contract labor at \$22 an hour, dividing \$1,760 by \$22 shows that 80 hours of contract services were utilized during this specific month (\$1,760 ÷ \$22 = 80 hours).

Total Productive Salaries and Wages. This figure, \$137,069, shows the combined amount of dollars paid for salaries, overtime, and contract labor during this month.

Overtime Premium. This shows the amount of dollars paid to personnel who worked overtime during this month. In most facilities overtime premium usually signifies funds paid to employees who worked a 12-hour shift. They receive 4 hours of overtime pay; the base rate of that 4 hours is included along with the regular salaries and wages; but this \$4,675 figure represents the overtime rate for those 4 hours.

Table 17-4 Monthly Operating Statement

Town and Country Hospital
Department: Medical-Surgical Units Combined*

	Actual	*Per Unit*	*Budget*	*Per Unit*
Unit of measure: pt. days	2,269		2,335	
Total revenue	$646,665	$285.00	$665,475	$285.00
Regular salaries and wages (with OT)	$135,309	$ 59.64	$137,830	$ 59.03
Contract	$ 1,760	$ 0.78	$ 10,000	$ 4.29
Total productive S & W	$137,069	$ 60.41	$147,830	$ 63.31
Overtime premium	$ 4,675	$ 2.06	$ 2,027	$ 0.87
Inservice/orientation	$ 7,529	$ 3.32	$ 9,648	$ 4.14
Vacation, holiday, sick	$ 24,258	$ 10.70	$ 24,258	$ 10.39
Total nonproductive S&W	$ 36,462	$ 16.07	$ 35,933	$ 15.39
Taxes and other benefits	$ 31,393	$ 13.84	$ 31,357	$ 13.43
Total S,W,& B	$204,924	$ 90.32	$215,120	$ 92.13
Medical supplies	$ 3,558	$ 1.57	$ 4,501	$ 1.93
Office supplies	$ 1,560	$ 0.69	$ 1,548	$ 0.67
Equipment lease/rental	$ 255	$ 0.12	$ 242	$ 0.11
Repair and maintenance	$ 50	$ 0.03	$ 72	$ 0.03
Travel/business meetings	$ 180	$ 0.08	$ 200	$ 0.09
Total other expense	$ 5,603	$ 2.47	$ 6,726	$ 2.88
Gross profit (loss)	$436,138	$192.22	$443,629	$190.00
Gross profit margin percent	68%		67%	

*Unit cost = Actual ÷ Patient days

Inservice/Orientation. This value refers to the amount of dollars paid to employees for either inservice or orientation time. In this example, totals for inservice and orientation equal $7,529.

Vacation, Holiday, Sick. This figure, $24,258, is the amount of dollars paid to the employees on the med-surg units for vacation time, holiday time, and sick time. Vacation and holiday time can be controlled only in that vacation time should be distributed evenly among employees and calendar months so that not all nursing personnel are absent from the unit at one time. Since holiday time is paid during the pay period in which it occurs, it is ideal to take time off for the holiday during the same period. However, vacation and holiday time are benefits paid and earned by the individual employee. Because they must be paid, one can monitor only how evenly vacation and holiday time are distributed. Sick time can be monitored and controlled to some degree. Nursing managers should document and monitor sick day patterns and follow up on individuals who have an excessive use of sick time. In this example, vacation, holiday, and sick time amounted to

$24,258. Nursing managers can further break down this amount of dollars by auditing the unit staffing records and time cards of their employees during this month to determine what portion of this amount was spent for vacation, for holiday, and for sick time.

Total Nonproductive Salaries and Wages. This figure indicates the combined amount of dollars spent on the overtime premium, inservice and orientation, vacation, holiday, and sick leave, that is, all nonproductive time. While the employee is on the premises and may be working during inservice or orientation, this time is actually considered nonproductive time because it may be only indirectly related to patient care. In Table 17-4 this figure equals $36,462.

Taxes and Other Benefits. This value of $31,393 refers to the amount of dollars paid to the employees on the medical/surgical units for taxes and other benefits such as medical insurance, dental insurance, life insurance, and pension plans.

Total Salaries, Wages, and Benefits. This is the grand total of salaries, wages, and benefits paid to the employees; it includes both productive and nonproductive salaries. Total salaries, wages, and benefits (SWB) in Table 17-4 amount to $204,924.

Medical Supplies. This refers to medical care materials and miscellaneous supplies purchased for the unit. This does not include the budgeted capital equipment but rather low-cost, necessary medical supplies such as a new IVAC thermometer, a portable patient scale, bedside bags, medicine cups, and other various nonpatient charge items. The medical supplies charged to the unit in Table 17-4 cost $3,558.

Office Supplies. Office supplies refers to the amount of dollars spent on paper items. This may include chart and requisition forms, depending on the facility. Office supplies could include a new pencil sharpener, staplers, paper clips, rubber bands, etc. Table 17-4 shows $1,560 for office supplies.

Equipment Lease/Rental. This indicates any items that may have been rented or leased for the med-surg unit during this month. Examples include the rental of a Clinitron bed and the lease of an electric typewriter. Table 17-4 shows $255 allocated for the lease or rental of special equipment.

Repair and Maintenance. This refers to the amount of dollars spent on repair or maintenance and charged to the unit. Depending on the facility, this may be either internally charged from the engineering department or externally charged from an outside contracted repair and maintenance service. Examples of this are repair of an electric bed and preventative maintenance or repair of a telemetry unit. In Table 17-4 such repairs and maintenances amounted to $50.

Travel/Business Meetings. This refers to the amount of dollars spent to send the unit managers or any members of the staff to lectures, seminars, or workshops held off of the hospital premises. In Table 17-4 this amounted to $180.

Total Other Expense. This is the combined total sum of the previous five categories, i.e., medical supplies, office supplies, equipment lease/rental, repair and maintenance, and travel/business meetings. In Table 17-4 this amount equals $5,603.

Gross Profit. The gross profit is determined by the amount of revenue ($646,665) less the expenses ($210,527). Another way to express gross profit as illustrated in Table 17-4 is as follows:

Revenue	$646,665
Expenses	− 210,527
Gross profit	$436,138

Gross Profit Margin Percentage. Gross profit margin percentage equals gross profit divided by total revenue. Another way to express this in Table 17-4 is as follows:

$$\text{gross profit margin percentage (68\%)} = \frac{\text{gross profit (\$436,138)}}{\text{total revenue (\$646,665)}}$$

Monthly Expense Report

The purpose of the monthly expense report is to provide each nursing unit manager with a clear picture of the amount of charges that it has actually incurred in comparison to its current budget. The nursing manager should be able to utilize this data as illustrated in Table 17-5 in order to account for each item and service charged to the department. If total dollar amounts do not agree, this discrepancy needs to be investigated by the manager. Vendor charges on the monthly expense report (Table 17-5) should in turn match the charges in the monthly operating statement (Table 17-4). For example, Table 17-5 states that $1,760 was paid to Kramer's Personnel Pool. The manager should first be able to verify that contract labor in this amount was utilized on the specific nursing unit by checking past staffing records. The nursing manager should multiply the recorded number of hours of contract labor times the hourly rate paid to the contracting agency. In this case if the contracting agency charged $22 an hour for a registered nurse, the nursing manager would expect to find 80 hours of contract service utilized during this month in question and documented in the staffing records ($1,760 ÷ 22 = 80). Second, the manager should be able to find and verify that expense on the monthly operating statement under the subtitle of contract labor.

Table 17-5 Monthly Expense Report

Town and Country Hospital — Month: *April 1983*
Department: Medical-Surgical Units Combined

	Vendor Number	*Vendor Name*	*Invoice Date*	*Invoice Amount*
1.	*Contract Labor*			
	K050642	Kramer's Personnel Pool	4-83	$1,760
2.	*Medical Supplies*			
	P121550	Daly Hospital Supply	3-83	390
	E082345	Marin Health Supplies	12-82	600
	J072272	J E H Supplies	3-83	207
	V110521	Medical Equipment by Kirby	11-82	2,200
	G120449	Gingers Health Supplies	3-83	161
3.	*Office Supplies*			
	H070641	M.E.H. Store Equipment	12-82	1,200
	M060751	Westlake Office Equipment	1-82	360
4.	*Equipment lease/rental*			
	R090432	Land-O-Nod Rentals	4-83	165
	I062909	Typewriters-R-Us	2-83	90
5.	*Repair and Maintenance*			
	C011581	C. Nicholas Repair & Maintenance	3-83	50
6.	*Travel/business meetings*			
	W061420	Mayfair Travel Agency	1-83	80
	B082646	DCRD and SFPD Airlines	3-83	100

NOTE

1. Beth Zaentz, Assistant Controller, Alta Bates Hospital, Berkeley, Calif.

Appendix 17-A

Self-Test of Operating Budget Statements

1. Indicate which of the following are productive hours (P) or nonproductive hours (NP).
   a) Working an 8-hour shift. __________
   b) Staying over 4 hours to cover the unit. __________
   c) Working on a holiday. __________
   d) A per-diem nurse working only half a shift. __________
   e) Being on call for 8 hours for the recovery room and not being called in.
   ____
   f) Being called by the nursing office to come to work the unit. You worked 6 hours, but were not really on call. __________
   g) Having the day off on the holiday itself. __________
   h) Being on call for 10 hours for the operating room. You were called in to work 4 hours. Is this all productive time? __________
   Explain:

2. Productive hours = __________ hours + __________ hours
   + __________ hours + __________ hours

Questions 3-5 refer to the labor hours report, Table 17-3.

3. On 1 South what were the overtime hours? __________
4. If 1 South showed 349 pt. days during this accounting period, what were the NHPPD on 1 South? __________

5. a) 1 South showed ________ inservice hours.
   b) How many FTEs does this figure reflect? ________
6. How do you calculate *paid* FTEs?

7. What is the unit of measure for the following departments/units?

Med-surg	________	CSR	________
ICU-CCU	________	Engineering	________
ER	________	Medical records	________
OR	________	Dietary	________

8. What does *unit cost* mean?

9. How is unit cost determined?

Questions 10-14 refer to the monthly operating statement, Table 17-4.

10. According to the monthly operating statement (Table 17-4), was VHS over or under budget for med-surg? ________
11. Can this be controlled? ________ How or how not?
12. Gross profit = ________ − ________.
13. Gross profit margin % = ________ ÷ ________.
14. Med-surg at Town and Country Hospital anticipated a total of ________ patient days. Instead, med-surg had ________ days. The actual patient days were ______ percent above or below budget?
15. a) What should happen to the med-surg unit cost?

    b) What should happen to the total department cost?

16. For which of the following should the supervisor/unit coordinator of a unit be held accountable?

Number of pts. budgeted?	________
Number of pts seen?	________
Total expenses?	________
Expenses per unit of measure?	________

ANSWERS TO SELF-TEST

1. a) P
   b) P
   c) P
   d) P
   e) NP
   f) P
   g) NP
   h) Only 4 hours are productive time. The on-call at home is nonproductive time.
2. Productive hours = regular hours + overtime hours + call-back hours + contract hours
3. On 1 South the overtime hours were 34.5 hours.
4. Total hours worked divided by patient days = nursing hours per patient day. 1,999.00 hours ÷ 349 patient days = 5.72 nursing hours per patient day.
5. a) 99 hours were allocated to inservice.
   b) This reflects 1.24 FTEs. 99.00 hours ÷ 80 hours (1 full-time equivalent) = FTEs
6. Total hours paid ÷ 80 = paid FTEs
7.

Med-Surg	patient days	CSR	items dispensed
ICU-CCU	patient days	Engineering	square feet of plant
ER	visits	Medical records	admissions/discharges
OR	cases	Dietary	meals served

8. Unit cost refers to the amount of dollars spent per unit of measure, i.e., patient days, patient visits, cases.
9. Unit cost is determined by the total amount of dollars spent divided by patient days (or unit of measure).
10. Total department cost for vacation, holiday, sick leave was exactly on budget. However, unit cost for vacation, holiday, sick leave was over budget. Unit cost should be the same as budget because total costs should be flexible as patient days decrease or increase.
11. Vacation time can be controlled only in that a great number of employees should not take vacation at the same time. Holiday time should be taken during the pay period in which it occurs so that employees do not accrue great amounts of holiday pay during nonholiday pay periods. Sick time can be controlled by monitoring, documenting, and following up on individuals who have excessive sick time.
12. Gross profit = total revenue − total expenses (SWB + expenses)
13. Gross profit margin % = gross profit ÷ revenue

14. The budget anticipated a total of 2,335 patient days. Instead this med-surg department had 2,269 patient days. The actual patient days on this unit were three percent *below* budget: 2,269 ÷ 2,335 = 97% of budgeted days met, therefore, 3 percent below budgeted days.
15. a) The med-surg *unit* cost should stay the same as budget because costs should flex as budgeted patient days increase or decrease.
    b) *Total* department cost should decrease by 3 percent.
16. A unit supervisor or unit coordinator can be partially accountable for the number of patients budgeted by assisting the controller with establishing a realistic budget based on trends, long-range strategic plans, and marketing plans for the area. The unit supervisor or unit coordinator is not accountable or responsible for the total number of patients seen since this is beyond control. She is responsible for total expenses of the department and accountable for expenses per unit of measure for the unit.

Chapter 18

The Challenge for Nursing Managers in the 1980s: Where Do We Go from Here?

OBJECTIVES

Following the completion of this chapter, the reader will be able to:

- list seven factors to consider when deciding staffing proportions of RNs, LVNs, and NAs and a desired type of nursing modality and
- develop an appreciation for the economics involved in making these decisions.

As hospital employees and as individuals with family and other responsibilities nurses are finding themselves in austere times. Medical economists speculate that one cause is the restricted attitude of the government toward health care. Health care, one of the largest businesses in America, will feel the impact and scars of the 1982 recession long after the economic wounds have healed. A primary challenge to hospital administrations is to develop policy and strategy to deal with and react intelligently to health care competition and the business side of health care: cost control, productivity, planning, and marketing. Hospital management teams need to develop hospitalwide action plans, recognizing that managers can't have everything that they want and recognizing the need to prioritize capital spending. Hospital management teams and hospital medical staffs need to work together as a professional group in order to implement a well-thought-out strategic business plan for the institution.[1]

As frequently happens when faced with stress, a person returns to basic roots, instincts, and basic needs. Thus for the nursing profession the economic crunch of health care has prompted nursing to remain committed toward its basic needs, primarily those of quality, accountability, and professional dedication. The dichotomy is centered around the environment with which nursing now has to contend in order to demonstrate that accountability and commitment. Nurses are being asked to exist with less dollars, less manpower, and often outmoded or less sophisticated equipment in a society with a rapidly advancing technology. Facing this dilemma, nurses need to maintain sight of three vital aspects of their professional commitment:

1. patient care and safety
2. professional job satisfaction
3. goals and philosophy of the institution and professional nursing practice

ISSUE OF COST EFFECTIVENESS

With increasing competition among health care delivery systems, hospitals, in order to survive, must deal not only with quality and accountability but also with the issues of consumer services and accessibility to health care. The future of health care delivery is directly contingent on the immediate implementation of cost-effective alternatives.

John C. Bedrosian, executive vice president of National Medical Enterprises in Los Angeles, spoke before the Hospital Association of Hawaii's annual meeting in November 1982. Mr. Bedrosian stressed that new measures are essential to avoid jeopardizing "the quality and the integrity of our health care delivery system in America." He added that hospital officials must recognize the current economic realities and support efforts to restrain the inflationary process affecting health care expenditures.

"Public awareness of spiraling health care costs is intensifying," Mr. Bedrosian said. "No one, including the government, wants a reduction in quality. They just want it for less, or to reduce their share of the cost.

"Today's, and most certainly tomorrow's, health care organization must be absolutely dedicated to delivering the most appropriate care in the least costly setting," he said. Budgets will be spread thinner and hospitals will need to become

> more efficient, more cost conscious, more competitive, and more innovative. Fiscal responsibility will be the primary consideration in the development of other innovative approaches to health care. If we do not shape the evolving mechanisms of health care, they will grind us into ineffectiveness.
>
> A truly competitive health care system is the best solution to maintain the quality of health care in America without further adding to the nation's economic woes.
>
> Unless something is done to relieve our growing capital prices, the quality and availability of health care across the nation will most certainly deteriorate. This financial shortage not only threatens our

> ability to expand capacity to keep pace with the accelerating demand, but prevents us from maintaining the system as it currently exists. Our ability to survive in the future then will be determined by our ability to be flexible and open minded.[2]

Each hospital facility should consider the most cost-effective delivery care method to meet its specific needs. Each hospital must also consider the impact of the following factors on the staffing proportions.

OTHER FACTORS

Hospital Location

A hospital located in a large metropolitan area where competition between hospitals is intense can experience competitive services and technology between facilities. Hospitals that offer renal or peritoneal dialysis services and sophisticated levels of critical care involving arterial lines and swanz ganz catheters require a continual upgrading and purchase of equipment with advanced interpretation abilities. The specialized skills of the RN/critical care nursing staff in turn require continuation of their educational development, which must enhance the standards of nursing practice along with the advancement of these critical care nursing skills.

Availability of Professional Nursing Staff

Consider the availability and access of professional nursing staff. Perhaps a rural facility may have difficulty recruiting and retaining experienced and qualified personnel. These facilities may need to justify the costs of elevated salaries to attract employees in addition to expensive recruitment tactics.

Philosophy of the Hospital—Service-Oriented or Care-Oriented

Let's discuss the issue of service versus care and how each is viewed by a hospital's medical staff, nursing staff, and patient populace. These two words have been used interchangeably and often with conflicting misinterpretation. Most hospital administrations can conduct a survey among patients to rate care. Nearly every patient will comment on:

- how promptly the call light was answered,
- whether the meals were served hot and on time, and whether the room was kept basically clean with bathroom facilities functioning properly and the room maintained at a comfortable temperature.

The patient is really making a judgment on:

- room service,
- meal service, and
- environmental services.

While the average patient may be evaluating service rather than care, this average patient can evaluate only what is seen. The patient probably cannot determine the quality of the EKGs read at the facility nor the speed at which the lab performs its tests and posts the results on patients' medical records. How many nursing administrators have ever heard a patient or family compliment the hospital on its comprehensive quality assurance plan or its low nosocomial infection rate? The average patient is not able to make a determination or judgment on most issues pertaining to care or quality of care. Rather the patient can judge, evaluate, and comment on issues of service.

The medical and nursing staff on the other hand may also be able to make some judgment on service as it is related to them by their patients. How many nursing administrators have experienced this scenario. Dr. Jones, chief of staff, comes into the office. While he may not appear angry, he has a displeased look on his face. He states, "My patient, Mrs. Germain, had to wait 35 minutes for her light to be answered last night before getting her hypo. I thought that the nursing care had improved."

Perhaps the nursing care has improved but the ability to deliver that care from a service standpoint may not live up to the ideal standards that nurses would like. An important distinction must be made: which is care and which is service? Which is more important? Is it more important that the nurse answer the light promptly (service) or administer the medication to the patient appropriately and in a safe manner by reviewing the pharmacological literature if necessary and watching for potential side effects (care)? Once again the handmaiden expectations of yesterday's nurse have resurfaced and crept their way into the clinical setting for today's professional nurse. The role of the nurse as the specialist or clinician remains in the background.

Service is not unimportant. Rather, there is a fine line between service and care; the two should not be confused in terms of evaluating performance as a nursing department responsible for providing that care and service.

Climate of the Medical Staff

A nursing administrator along with the hospital administrator should explore the stages of the development and growth of the medical staff in the facility. A medical staff that chooses to become involved in the running of a nursing department will clearly impact the nursing administration.

As pointed out in Chapter 4, in many facilities physicians choose to participate in the superficial manipulation of management affairs of the nursing department rather than allow management to function under the auspices of the nursing administration. The most reliable solutions and alternatives are the direct result of joint nurse/physician/administrator efforts. Lack of support of the hospital and nursing administration by a physician, or even worse by a group of physicians, can have a dramatically negative effect.

The frequency of complaints with regard to nursing care offered by the medical staff and the mechanism whereby these complaints are registered affects to some degree the difficulty that the nursing administration faces in developing its own systems. If the medical staff chooses to vocalize concerns of poor care or insufficient staff at such inappropriate times as committee meetings, the results can, and often do, have a contagious effect among other committee members. If some physicians distastefully and frequently register blatant complaints publicly at committee meetings with the desired action then taken by the administration—such as the termination of a nursing employee based on the physician's outrage—other physicians can interpret this as an acceptable behavior and a mechanism to get what they want. The accepted behavior exhibited in any group is dictated by the outcome of that behavior.

Costs of Staffing Complements

In many hospitals and nursing administrations frequent discussion regards the controversy of an all-RN staff as opposed to some acceptable complement of RN and LVN staff. The nursing literature is saturated with articles on the expenditures of an all-RN staff compared to a staff consisting of ratios of RNs and LVNs. Many nursing management textbooks refer to various models that can be utilized and implemented by staff nursing units. But staffing involves more than a simple numbers game. Proper staffing should allow for an appropriate mix of personnel based on such factors as patient acuity and total unit acuity. Long-range nurse satisfaction is the end result when nursing personnel are appropriately placed in positions for which they have been adequately oriented, inserviced, and prepared. Each facility must independently decide, after comprehensive research, whether an all-RN staff is feasible from a cost-effective perspective in addition to the realistic application from a productive standpoint.

Initially an all RN-staff can be a somewhat more expensive investment than a staff complement of RNs and LVNs, and perhaps NAs; in the long run it may prove more cost effective. For example, in the authors' facility the past practice among the LVN personnel did not allow them to give medications or regulate IV therapy. Because of an extreme shortage of RNs, the nursing management decided that the LVN group should receive proper orientation, inservice, and certification in medication administration and IV procedures in accordance with the legal guidelines established for an LVN in the state of California. A great deal of time and money went into achieving the goal of educating and orienting the LVNs. This specific facility employed 37 LVNs. A 32-hour course was developed for medication administration. The administrative cost therefore to send each LVN to this class was 32 hours times $9.72, the average salary for an LVN in this facility. This investment totaled $311.04 for each LVN to attend the medication administration class; this totaled $11,508.48 to send the 37 LVNs through the class. The medication classes were gradually conducted over one year. Not included in this figure is the amount of dollars spent for benefits paid to these 37 LVNs and the salaries for the inservice educators to train the LVNs for medication administration as well as their course preparation time.

While this is an impressive expenditure, nursing administrations need to go one step further to justify the outcome of this cost. For example, in the state of California, an LVN is required to have 30 units of continuing education classes over a two-year period. While there was a cost to the hospital to conduct the course, the course helped the LVNs to meet the state requirements for CE credits. This was a major motivator for the LVNs to enroll in the class. This method accomplished a two-fold achievement. First, upgrading the level of practice of the LVN resulted in a more productive work force; second, the 30 units of CE classes were controlled by the nursing administration, which forced utilization of educational leave for appropriate courses. This is an excellent method to pave the way for more productive staff yet minimize the expense of the all-RN staff concept.

IMPACT OF CLASSIFICATION AND STAFFING SYSTEMS

Patient classification systems and nurse staffing systems are as numerous and ever-changing as the individuals in a nursing department who create them. To develop effectively and maintain strategic systems with patient classification as a measurement and tool for the system, nursing administrators must ask a number of questions about the desired goal. There are numerous reasons, and quite legitimate ones, why structured systems are needed for nurse staffing: regulatory requirements, both state and federal; guidelines for management; definition for staff nurse; etc. Probably the primary justification for structured systems is that gray and difficult-to-measure area called quality, accountability, and professional commitment.

The nursing profession, like many other professions, has periods of crisis when its principles are scrutinized. With dramatic nursing shortages the challenge to the nursing profession to meet its goals of quality and accountability has become even more threatened. Some current writers even proclaim nursing as a dying profession and suggest that nursing is commiting suicide because of its lack of organization and its continual wallowing in images of the past, those of subservience and servitude. To survive in the 1990s, nursing must seek new and innovative methods to ensure continued ability to provide its highest service, that of quality patient care and safety to the consumer.

Scott Gross, senior vice president, south central region of National Medical Enterprises, spoke at the annual meeting of Nursing Administrators of National Medical Enterprises. Mr. Gross, an advocate for the nursing profession for the 1980s, emphasized that most hospital administrators, physicians, and nursing personnel would agree that the quality of care in a hospital is influenced primarily by the quality of medical care and the quality of nursing care given in the hospital. For the most part patients receive nursing care above and beyond anything else in the hospital. A patient day consists of 24 hours. With the exception of approximately 20 minutes that the physician will spend with a patient and approximately 20 minutes that allied health professionals spend with the patient, the remaining 23 hours and 20 minutes is predominantly the responsibility of the nursing department.[3]

Mr. Gross also agreed that in some facilities there is an archaic attitude toward nursing and a historic lack of recognition for the roles that a nurse plays in the management team. More than ever before what is necessary during the 1980s is to put the professional back into the nurse. In order to do this, nursing departments and nurses themselves must play a greater role in the decision making and development of health care policy in the hospital. In order to make this happen, the nursing profession must recognize the unique needs of the professional nurse. These needs may be in areas such as financial, professional growth and achievement, and educational assistance. An environment where a nurse receives not only financial rewards for work but also professional satisfaction must be created. The environment must allow nurses to receive growth and opportunity in the leadership and management roles in nursing departments. Professional nurses need the opportunity to grow and attain satisfaction in their environment. Of primary importance is creating a structure within hospitals to make growth and professional satisfaction a reality.

The nursing profession is faced with major challenges in the 1980s. Cost cutting and governmental changes in reimbursement policies will have a dramatic impact on the ability of a hospital to stay viable financially and to deliver services to the patient. The 1990s will bring a level of cost consciousness far beyond anything in the past. The nursing profession has a challenge, a challenge to find ways to continue to maintain and improve the quality of care that nurses give patients and to do so as economically as possible. Nursing management teams must unleash the creative forces within themselves to develop alternatives and discover better ways to deliver that care to patients.

Nurses must speak up. Through individuals or through local hospitals nursing management must speak out and participate in the establishment of policy as it relates to nursing. Many new things will happen to nursing in the 1990s and roles will change. No one has to put any limits on nurses or their role. There is a shortage of people in the world who desire to make that commitment both in terms of quantity and quality to meet the needs of the health care industry today and in the future.[4] If nursing managers want to be a part of the great challenges that face them in the 1990s, they must make that commitment and become contributing members of the change process.

NOTES

1. John P. Rinset, vice president, hospital operations, northwest region, National Medical Enterprises, Modesto, California, from a speech before the Board of Directors, Doctors Hospital of Pinole, February 16, 1983, Pinole, CA.
2. John C. Bedrosian, executive vice president, National Medical Enterprises, Inc., speech before the annual meeting of the Hospital Association of Hawaii, Honolulu, November 1982.
3. Scott Gross, senior vice president, south central region, National Medical Enterprises, speech before Nursing Administrators Meeting, New Orleans, November 1981.
4. Ibid.

Appendix A

Suggested Readings

BOOKS

Althaus, Joan Nietz; Hardyck, Nancy McDonald; Pierce, Patricia Blair; and Rodgers, Marilyn S. *Nursing Decentralization: The El Camino Experience*. Rockville, Md.: Aspen Systems Corporation, 1981.

Bauer, Raymond A., and Gergen, Kenneth J., eds. *The Study of Policy Formation*. New York: The Free Press, 1968.

Berman, Edgar. *The Solid Gold Stethoscope*. New York: Macmillan Publishing Co., Inc., 1976.

Berman, Howard J., and Weeks, Lewis E. *The Financial Management of Hospitals*. 3d ed. Ann Arbor, Mich.: Health Administration Press, 1978.

Bormann, Ernest G., and Bormann, Nancy C. *Effective Small Group Communication*. 2d ed. Minneapolis: Burgess Publishing Company, 1976.

Brown, Barbara J., ed. *Nurse Staffing: A Practical Guide*. Rockville, Md.: Aspen Systems Corporation, 1980.

Dale Carnegie and Associates. *Managing through People*. New York: Simon and Schuster, 1978.

Department of Health, Education and Welfare. *Methods for Studying Nurse Staffing in a Patient Unit*. Health Resources Administration. HEW Publication no. HRA78-3. Hyattsville, Md.: Public Health Service, 1978.

Di Vincenti, Marie. *Administering Nursing Service*. Boston: Little, Brown & Company, 1977.

Ehrlich, Nathaniel, J. *Psychology and Contemporary Affairs*. Monterey, Calif.: Brooks/Cole Publishing Company, 1972.

Ewing, David, W. *Freedom Inside the Organization*. New York: McGraw-Hill Paperbacks, 1977.

Filoromo, Tina, and Ziff, Dolores. *Nurse Recruitment: Strategies for Success*. Rockville, Md.: Aspen Systems Corporation, 1980.

Galbraith, Joy. *Designing Complex Organizations*. Reading, Mass.: Addison-Wesley Publishing Company, 1973.

Ganong, Joan M., and Ganong, Warren L. *Nursing Management*. Rockville, Md.: Aspen Systems Corporation, 1980.

Gellerman, Saul W. *The Management of Human Relations*. Hinsdale, Ill.: Dryden Press, 1966.

Goldhaber, Gerald M. *Organizational Communication*. Dubuque, Iowa: Wm. C. Brown Company, 1974.

Grissum, Marlene, and Spengler, Carol. *Woman Power and Health Care*. Boston: Little, Brown & Company, 1976.

Grossman, Lee. *The Change Agent*. New York: Anacom, 1974.

Hackman, J. Richard, and Suttle, J. Lloyd. *Improving Life at Work: Behavioral Science Approaches to Organizational Change*. Santa Monica, Calif.: Goodyear Publishing Company, Inc., 1977.

Jantsch, Erich. *Design for Evolution: Self-Organization and Planning in the Life of Human Systems*. New York: George Braziller, Inc., 1975.

Jun, Jong, S., and Storm, William B. *Tomorrow's Organizations: Challenges and Strategies*. Glenview, Ill., and Brighton, England: Scott, Foresman and Company, 1973.

Kanter, Rosabeth Moss. *Men and Women of the Corporation*. New York: Basic Books, Inc., 1977.

Kolin, Philip C., and Kolin, Janeen L. *Professional Writing for Nurses in Education, Practice, and Research*. St. Louis: C.V. Mosby Company, 1980.

Kramer, Marlene, and Schmalenberg, Claudia. *Path to Biculturalism*. Rockville, Md.: Aspen Systems Corporation, 1977.

Leavitt, Harold, J.; Dill, William R.; and Eyring, Harry B. *The Organizational World*. New York: Harcourt Brace Jovanovich, Inc., 1973.

Lewis, Charles E.; Fein, Roshi; and Mechanic, David. *A Right to Health: The Problem of Access to Primary Medical Care*. New York: John Wiley & Sons, 1976.

May, Rollo. *Man's Search for Himself*. New York: Dell Publishing, Co., Inc., 1953.

May, Rollo. *Power and Innocence*. New York: Dell Publishing Co., Inc., 1972.

Michael, Donald N. *On Learning to Plan—and Planning to Learn*. San Francisco, Washington, and London: Jossey-Bass Publishers, 1978.

O'Toole, James. *Work and the Quality of Life*. Cambridge, Mass., and London: The M.I.T. Press, 1974.

Pugh, D.S., ed. *Organizational Theory*. Harmondsworth, Middlesex, England: Penguin Books, Ltd., 1971.

Somers, Anne R., and Somers, Herman M. *Health and Health Care: Policies in Perspective*. Rockville, Md.: Aspen Systems Corporation, 1977.

Stevens, Barbara J. *The Nurse as Executive*. 2d ed. Rockville, Md.: Aspen Systems Corporation, 1980.

Vast, Carolyn, L. *The Burnt-out Administrator*. New York: Springer Publishing Company, 1980.

Work in America. Report of a Special Task Force to the Secretary of Health, Education, and Welfare. Prepared under the auspices of the W.E. Upjohn Institute for Employment Research. Cambridge, Mass. and London, England: The M.I.T. Press, 1976.

Wright, Robert Grandford. *The Nature of Organizations*. Encino, Calif.: Dickenson Publishing Company, Inc., 1977.

PERIODICALS AND JOURNALS

Althaus, Joan Nietz; Hardyck, Nancy McDonald; Pierce, Patricia Blair; and Rodgers, Marilyn S. "Nurse Staffing in a Decentralized Organization, Part I." *Journal of Nursing Administration* 12, no. 3 (March 1982): 34–39.

Althaus, Joan Nietz; Hardyck, Nancy McDonald; Pierce, Patricia Blair; and Rodgers, Marilyn S. "Decentralized Budgeting: Holding the Purse Strings, Part I." *Journal of Nursing Administration* 12, no. 5 (May 1982): 15–20.

Barhan, Virginia, and Schneider, William R. "MARTRIX: A Unique Patient Classification System." *Journal of Nursing Administration,* December 1980, pp. 25–35.

Bell, R. "Diagnosing Nursing Costs." *Cost Containment Newsletter* 22, no. 10 (October 1982): pp. 3–7.

British Medical Journal. "Changing Relations between Doctors and Nurses." October 16, 1982, pp. 1130–32.

Bronstein, Jean E., and Walker, Duane D. "Developing a Patient Classification System. On the Scene: Stanford University Hospital," *Nursing Administration Quarterly* 5 (Winter 1981): pp. 17–21.

Cassell, Rebecca, and Shilling, Mary. "Study Projects Nursing Staff Needs, Budget." *Hospitals,* July 17, 1979, pp. 108, 114, 118, 122.

Castledine, G. "Planning the Patients' Progress." *Nursing Mirror* 150, no. 13 (March 27, 1980): 12.

Chen, Martin K., and Yang, Grace L. "A Quantitative Index for Evaluating Patient Care with Longitudinal Data." *International Journal of Epidemiology* 8, no. 3 (1979): 265–70.

Chin, Ying-Hsin. "Planning Hospital Nursing Units for Patient Care." *Bull. N.Y. Aca. Med.*, March 1981, pp. 144–148.

Cochran, Jeannette. "Refining A Patient-Acuity System over Four Years." *Hospital Progress*, February 1979, pp. 56–60.

Cohen, Adrene G. "Putting Together an Applicable Patient Categorization System for a Hospital and Nursing Home." *Hospital Topics*, May/June 1981, pp. 16–21.

Daubert, Elizabeth A. "Patient Classification System and Outcome Criteria." *Nursing Outlook*, July 1979, pp. 450–454.

Davis, Lola A. "How Do You Follow Up? *Journal of Nursing Administration*, February 1980, pp. 25–30.

Giovannetti, Phyllis. "Understanding Patient Classification Systems." *Journal of Nursing Administration*, February 1979, pp. 4–9.

Hanna, Diane L. "Rx for Reality Shock: A Care Plan for the New Nurse." *Miss RN*, June 1981, pp. 9–11.

Higgerson, Nancy J., and Vanslyck, Ann. "Variable Billing for Services: New Fiscal Direction for Nursing." *Journal of Nursing Administration*, June 1982, pp. 20–27.

Holle, Mary Lou. "Staffing: What the Books Don't Tell You." *Nursing Management*, March 1982, pp. 14–16.

Jackson, Bettie S., and Resnick, Joan. "Comparing Classification Systems." *Nursing Management*, November 1982, pp. 13–19.

Kanter, Rosabeth Moss. "The Middle Manager as Innovator." *Harvard Business Review*, July/August 1982, pp. 95–105.

Knaus, William A.; Zimmerman, Jack E.; Wagner, Douglas P.; Draper, Elizabeth A.; and Lawrence, Diane E. "APACHE—Acute Physiology and Chronicle Health Evaluation: A Physiologically Based Classification System." *Critical Care Medicine*, August 1981, pp. 591–597.

Kushner, Tricia D. "The Nursing Profession: Condition: Critical." *Ms* 11, no. 2 (August 1973): 72–102.

Lavery, William J.; Maynard, William C.; and Ivan, Judy. "Accountability Study Focuses on Staff Abilities and Patient Needs." *Michigan Hospital*, October 1979, pp. 26–29.

LaViolette, Suzanne. "Classification Systems Remedy Billing Inequity." *Modern Healthcare*, September 1979, pp. 32–33.

Lewis, Kaye. "What Organized Nursing Expects." *Hospital Administration in Canada*, July 1976, pp. 23–24.

Main, Jeremy. "Hard Times Catch Up with Executives." *Fortune*, September 20, 1982, pp. 50–54.

Manthey, Marie. "A Theoretical Framework for Primary Nursing." *Journal of Nursing Administration,* June 1980, pp. 11–16.

McCullock, Sybil. "Designing a Nursing Care Plan." *Australian Nurses' Journal,* November 1980, p. 14.

Mendenhall, Robert C.; Lewis, Charles E.; DeFlorio, George P.; and Girard, Roger A. "A National Study of Medical and Surgical Specialties." *Journal of the American Medical Association,* May 18, 1979, pp. 2180–85.

Modrow, Robert, and Luke, Roice D. "The 'New' Accountability and the Role of the Nurse Administrator." *Hospital Forum,* November/December 1979, pp. 13–14.

Mohney, Sandra J. "Why Participative Management in the Modern Hospital?" *Supervisor Nurse,* May 1980, pp. 36–38.

"New Nurse Program Lowers Turnover." *Hospital,* August 16, 1981, p. 60.

Osinski, Elsie G., and Powals, Jill G. "The Cost of All R.N. Staffed Primary Nursing." *Supervisor Nurse,* January 1980, pp. 16–20.

Peterson, Carol J. "The New Nurse and the New Physician." *Annals of Internal Medicine* 96, no. 3 (March 1982): 374.

Reinert, Pamela, and Grant, Donald R. "A Classification System to Meet Today's Needs." *Journal of Nursing Administration,* January 1981, pp. 21–25.

Roehrl, Patricia K. "Patient Classification: A Pilot Test." *Supervisor Nurse,* February 1979, pp. 21–27.

Rotkovitch, Rachel. "The Nursing Director's Role in Money Management." *Journal of Nursing Administration,* November/December 1981, pp. 13–16.

Schneider, Don. "An Ambulatory Care Classification System: Design, Development and Evaluation." *Health Service Research* 14(1979): 76–87.

Simendinger, Earl A., and Gilbert, Vicki. "Flexible Staffing." *Supervisor Nurse,* March 1979, pp. 43–46.

Skinner, Wickham. "Big Hat, No Cattle: Managing Human Resources, Part I." *Journal of Nursing Administration* 12, nos. 7-8 (July and August 1982): 27–29.

Skinner, Wickham. "Big Hat, No Cattle: Managing Human Resources, Part II." *Journal of Nursing Administration* 12, no. 9 (September 1982): 32–35.

Spitzer, Roxane. "The Nurse in the Corporate World." *Supervisor Nurse,* April 1981, pp. 21–24.

"Staffing Patterns in Medical and Surgical Units." *Hospitals,* Journal of the American Hospital Association, January 1, 1979, pp. 29–30.

Thomas, Debbie. "Medical-Surgical Nursing Practice Standards: Standard V: The Plan for Nursing Care Is Implemented." *Oklahoma Nurse,* March 1981.

Weisman, Carol S. "Recruit from Within: Hospital Nurse Retention in the 1980's." *Journal of Nursing Administration* 12, no. 5 (May 1982): 24–31.

Wellever, Anthony. "Variance Analysis: A Tool for Cost Control." *Journal of Nursing Administration* 12, nos. 7-8 (July-August 1982): 23–26.

White, Charles H., and Mahan, Paul B. "Nursing: A Part-time Profession?" *CHA Insight,* November 12, 1981, pp. 1–4.

Youell, Linda. "Patient Classification Program." *Dimensions in Health Services,* November 1979, pp. 17–18.

Young, Wanda W.; Swinkola, Robert B.; and Hutton, Martha A. "Assessment of the AUTOGRP Patient Classification System." *Medical Care,* February 1980, pp. 228–44.

Appendix B

Other Resources

Norma Anderson Badger, RN, BSW
Coordinator, Utilization Review and Discharge Planning
Doctors Hospital of Pinole
Pinole, California

John C. Bedrosian
Executive Vice President
National Medical Enterprises
Los Angeles, California

Shirley Campanile
Associate Administrator
Doctors Hospital of Pinole
Pinole, California

Scott Gross
Senior Vice President
South Central Region
National Medical Enterprises
New Orleans, Louisiana

Frankie Nail, RN, MN
Assistant Administrator
Nursing Services
Jo Ellen Smith and F. Edward Hebert Hospitals
New Orleans, Louisiana

John P. Rinset
Vice President
Hospital Operations, Northwest Region
National Medical Enterprises
Modesto, California

Beth Zaentz
Assistant Controller
Alta Bates Hospital
Berkeley, California

Index*

A

* Page numbers in italics represent art work (tables, figures etc.)

E

F

G

H

About the Authors

Elizabeth Nancy Lewis has been an assistant administrator, nursing services, in acute care facilities since 1977. She has had extensive experience in clinical nursing practice in the areas of general medicine, surgery, obstetrics, operating room, critical care, and inservice education. Ms. Lewis earned her RN from St. Barnabas Hospital School of Nursing, Minneapolis; BS, Nursing Administration, from the University of Minnesota; and MS, Health Services Administration, and PhD, Health Services Administration, from Golden Gate University and Columbia Pacific University. She is certified in nursing administration through the American Nurses' Association and is a member of the American Society of Nursing Service Administrators.

Patricia Vince Carini has been a head nurse and quality assurance coordinator and has been responsible for nursing supervision and nurse recruitment. She has had experience in clinical nursing practice in medical and surgical nursing as well as in developing nurse staffing patterns and position control programs. Ms. Carini earned a BSN from San Francisco State University and an MPA from Hayward State University.